Your Body Can Heal Itself

Over 87 Foods Everyone Should Eat

Publisher's Note

The editors of FC&A have taken careful measures to ensure the accuracy and usefulness of the information in this book. While every attempt was made to assure accuracy, some Web sites, addresses, telephone numbers, and other information may have changed since printing.

This book is intended for general information only. It does not constitute medical advice or practice. We cannot guarantee the safety or effectiveness of any treatment or advice mentioned. Readers are urged to consult with their health care professionals and get their approval before undertaking therapies suggested by information in this book, keeping in mind that errors in the text may occur as in all publications and that new findings may supersede older information.

"Draw close to God, and God will draw close to you."

James 4:8

Contents

■ ■ ■ ■ ■ ■ ■ ■ ■ ■ ■ ■ ■

20 take-charge tactics for super health

Score big with vitamin-packed veggies

Fruit: sweet treats yield big rewards

Harvest the goodness of whole grains

Beef up your protein with beans and legumes

Nuts & Seeds: small but mighty

Anti-aging power from the sea

Punch up your diet with low-fat dairy

Quick guide: nutrition by condition

Contents

20 take-charge tactics for super health

1 *Separate good carbs from bad*

It's time to stop depriving yourself. "Carb" is not a four-letter word. It's the fuel that makes your body go. The key to staying healthy and slimming down is not to cut them from your diet — it's to eat the right ones.

Carbohydrates fill up your tank with most of the energy you need every day, not to mention vitamins, minerals, and fiber. In fact, lots of healthy foods, including cereal, fruit, starchy vegetables, and even milk, contain carbs.

Scientists classify carbs as either complex or simple. Starch and fiber are complex. Sugars, like lactose in milk and fructose in fruits, are simple. For a long time, people thought simple carbs were bad for you and complex carbs were good. Now all carbohydrates are getting a bad rap, thanks to the low-carb diet craze. Neither is true. Confused? Don't worry — finding "good" carbs is as easy as 1-2-3.

Eat nutrient-dense foods. Some high-carb foods are more nutritious than others. A Twinkie has the same amount of carbohydrates as a cup of fresh orange juice, but guess which one is better for you?

When you drink orange juice, you're not just getting empty carbs. You're getting vitamin C and potassium, plus the B-vitamins folate and thiamin. Twinkies, on the other hand, are not nutrient-dense. They fill you up with sugar and fat but virtually no vitamins, minerals, or fiber. Choose carb-containing foods that give you lots of nutrients, and you'll get more bang for your buck.

Pick unprocessed foods. Don't think of carbs as simple versus complex. Instead, think refined versus unrefined.

- Foods containing refined carbohydrates have gone through more processing, which tends to strip them of their nutrients. And the more refined a carbohydrate, the faster its sugars get into your bloodstream. White flour, white bread, and white rice are examples of refined carbohydrates.

■ The less processed the food, the less refined the carbs. Whole-wheat breads, brown rice, whole beans, and fresh vegetables are minimally processed, so they're as close to natural as can be. That means they keep more of their original nutrients and digest more slowly, so their sugars enter your bloodstream gradually instead of in a rush.

Why does it matter if a carb is refined or unrefined? Here's why. Many studies link refined carbohydrates with the development of chronic diseases, such as type 2 diabetes and cardiovascular disease, which includes heart disease, stroke, and heart attack. Eating lots of refined carbs tends to raise your triglycerides, lower your "good" HDL cholesterol, and wreak havoc on blood sugar and insulin levels.

Chow down on whole grains. While you're at it, make those unprocessed foods you're eating whole grain. A kernel of wheat has three edible parts.

■ The germ, the tiny wheat seed, sits in the center of the kernel and is rich in vitamins and minerals.

■ The endosperm is the soft, white part that surrounds the germ. It contains starch and protein.

■ Bran is the protective coating around the kernel, like the shell of a nut. It's loaded with fiber and nutrients.

Whole-grain foods are made using the entire wheat kernel — all three edible parts. This means they pack a huge nutritional wallop. Refined-grain foods, like white and unbleached flour, are made using only the endosperm, so they're mostly starch and little else.

At least half the grains you eat every day should be whole grains. Add up the scientific evidence, and you'll discover they may lower your risk for heart disease, digestive cancers, diabetes, and diverticulosis. You'll learn how to spot whole-grain foods by reading *Get a handle on food labels* in this section. For help buying healthy breads, check out *Basic rules for buying healthier breads* in the Grains chapter.

2 *Feel better with fiber*

If eating one thing could lower your cholesterol, help you lose weight, protect you from diabetes and colon cancer, and keep you regular, wouldn't you eat it?

Fiber can do all of this and more. It's the part of a plant your body can't digest. It gives leaves, stems, and seeds their shape and a stalk of celery its stiffness. Best of all, it boasts loads of healing properties.

There are two main types of fiber — soluble and insoluble — each with their own health benefits. A food may contain more of one than the other, but most foods offer a mixture of both.

- Soluble. This type of fiber dissolves in water, where it forms a gel. Soluble fibers include pectin in fruits, which makes jellies gel; gums, which thicken salad dressings; psyllium seed husks; and beta glucan in oats and barley.

- Insoluble. This is the kind of fiber you imagine when you think of "roughage." It absorbs water without dissolving the way soluble fiber does. Lignans in whole-grain foods; cellulose in cereal brans, fruits, and vegetables; and resistant starch in beans, lentils, and barley are all insoluble fibers.

These two types of fiber have some amazing effects inside your body, giving you the power to slim down and win the battle against major diseases.

Lose weight. Your body can't digest fiber, so you don't get any energy from it. That makes it the original zero-calorie snack. Because it adds bulk, high-fiber foods can help you feel fuller with fewer calories, making them a dieter's dream.

Lower cholesterol. Your liver turns cholesterol in your blood into the digestive juice bile. Soluble fibers, such as pectin and beta glucan, grab onto this bile-cholesterol in your intestines and carry it out of your body, along with stool. Your liver then has to pull more cholesterol from your blood to make more bile. The result — a drop in blood cholesterol levels.

Soothe digestive problems. Fiber softens stool for easier passage and bulks it up so it moves faster through your digestive tract. Put it all together, and fiber relieves constipation, prevents hemorrhoids, and lowers your risk of diverticulosis and appendicitis. Pectin may also soothe the symptoms of irritable bowel syndrome and Crohn's disease, while psyllium could help reduce flare-ups from ulcerative colitis.

Dodge diabetes. The soluble fiber in foods like beans and oats helps prevent and control type 2 diabetes by dampening blood sugar and insulin spikes after meals. Soluble fiber slows your digestion of carbohydrates, so you absorb their sugar more slowly into your bloodstream.

Clobber cancer. In general, insoluble fiber speeds up the movement of food through your digestive tract, which whisks cancer-causing compounds out of your colon before they do harm. Plus, the breakdown of resistant starch in your colon produces an anti-colon-cancer compound called butyric acid. Lignans may also slash your risk of breast, ovarian, colon, and prostate cancers by blocking the action of estrogen in these cells.

The National Academy of Sciences, which sets the Dietary Reference Intakes (DRI) for nutrients, says women over the age of 50 should eat at least 21 grams (g) of fiber each day. Men over age 50 should aim for 30 g daily.

Most people only get about half of that, even though fiber is everywhere. In fact, some of the least expensive foods, like beans, are among the best sources. The American Dietetic Association says, if you eat 2,000 calories a day, you can meet your fiber goals by eating at least:

- 4 1/2 cups of fruits and vegetables each day.
- 3 ounces of whole-grain foods daily.
- 3 cups of legumes a week.

Add high-fiber foods to your diet gradually to give your system time to adjust. Upping your fiber intake too fast can cause gas and bloating. Be sure to drink plenty of fluids, too, to help move all that fiber smoothly through your digestive tract.

3 *Satisfy a sweet tooth*

Americans eat, on average, nearly half a pound of sugar every day, mostly from products like sodas made with added sugar. People get 25 percent of their daily calories from sugars like these, even though experts warn only 10 percent of your daily calories should come from sugar.

It's serious business. Too much sugar seems to wreak havoc in your body, raising your triglycerides and lowering your "good" HDL cholesterol. So what's a sweet tooth to do? Never fear. Indulging doesn't have to mean harming your health.

Dip into honey. Table sugar, honey, molasses, brown sugar, raw sugar — which one is better for you? They all have roughly the same calories and carbohydrates per teaspoon, and some contain vitamins, minerals, or fiber. Honey, however, boasts healthful plant compounds, including antioxidants, the others don't. Plus, it's sweeter than table sugar, so you can use less and get the same taste.

Stir honey into warm milk, and you get a delicious three-in-one folk remedy for soothing a sore throat, stopping a cough, and helping you sleep. Some people say honey even eases arthritis pain. And many kinds of honey act as a natural antibiotic, battling infection and healing minor wounds.

Steer clear of added sugar. From baked goods to sodas, cooks and food manufacturers alike love to add sugar to food. Unfortunately, diets high in added sugar contribute to obesity and increase your risk for pancreatic cancer and tooth decay.

If you're over the age of 55, most of your added sugar probably comes from cookies and cakes, followed closely by table sugar, syrup, candy, jams, and jellies; nondiet colas, ginger ale, and root beer; and milk products, including ice cream, sweetened yogurt, and chocolate milk. Check the ingredient list on a food's label and avoid treats where sugar is the first or second ingredient.

Speed healing with sugar

Honey is an old folk remedy for healing cuts and scrapes, but a paste of sugar and water may also do the trick. Sugar works by pulling water out of a wound. That may battle infecting bacteria, help remove dirt, and even reduce scarring. Use regular granulated sugar and just enough water to form a paste. But be careful — sugar can affect your blood's ability to clot. Wait a day after the bleeding stops before you try this remedy.

Find alternatives to fructose. This type of sugar naturally occurs in healthy foods like fruits and honey, but manufacturers tweak it to make it sweeter, then add this super-sugar to food during processing. The result — a recipe for disaster.

Research links added fructose to metabolic syndrome, hardening of the arteries, cardiovascular disease, and liver disease. Baked goodies, frozen foods, nondiet sodas, fruit drinks, candies, syrups, and condiments are prime sources of added fructose. Check ingredient labels and limit foods that contain high-fructose corn syrup or crystalline fructose.

Switch to artificial. If you can't beat your craving for sugary snacks, consider those made with artificial sweeteners.

- Reduced-calorie sweeteners, or sugar alcohols, pack about half the calories and carbs as regular sugar. You'll often see them in "sugar-free" and "no sugar added" products, but beware — they can still raise your blood sugar. This group includes all the "ols" — mannitol, sorbitol, xylitol, lactitol, erythritol, and maltitol — as well as isomalt and hydrogenated starch hydrolysates.

- Low-calorie sweeteners have no calories and no carbs and won't raise your blood sugar. Sucralose (SPLENDA), aspartame (Equal,

NutraSweet), saccharin (Sweet 'N Low, Sugar Twin), and acesulfame potassium (Sweet One, Swiss Sweet, Sunett) all belong to this exclusive club.

Concerns have dogged aspartame over its potential to cause cancer. The Food and Drug Administration has looked at over 100 studies and declared it safe for people to use. It can, however, trigger headaches in some people. If you're one of them, consider sweetening with sucralose (SPLENDA) instead.

4 *Pile on plant foods*

Fruits, vegetables, legumes, nuts, seeds, whole grains, green tea, dark chocolate, and wine — all of these plant foods contain special disease-fighting compounds called phytochemicals. Your body doesn't need phytochemicals to survive the way it does vitamins, minerals, and other nutrients, but they can help you live longer and fight off chronic diseases.

Discover the root of many maladies. As your cells burn energy, they create leftover compounds known as free radicals — very unstable molecules that damage the genetic material, or DNA, inside your cells. Since you constantly churn out free radicals, it's no surprise how much damage they end up doing. Scientists estimate your cells suffer 10,000 free radical attacks every day.

Mostly, your cells fix themselves. Over time, they simply can't keep up, and DNA damage accumulates. Free radicals also attack and oxidize LDL cholesterol, which can lead to plaque buildup in your arteries. All in all, experts finger free radical damage as a major culprit in cancer, atherosclerosis, Alzheimer's disease, Parkinson's disease, mental decline, cataracts, arthritis, immune problems, and emphysema and other lung diseases.

Protect your cells to prevent disease. That's where loading your plate with plants comes in. Some phytochemicals act as antioxidants, supercharged compounds that team up with your body's natural defenses to stop thuggish free radicals from forming and disarm them before they wreak havoc on your cells. Certain nutrients, including the mineral selenium and vitamins A, C, E, and beta carotene, also act as antioxidants in your body.

Years of study show eating plenty of fruits and vegetables helps you live longer and prevent disease. Experts think the hundreds of antioxidants in these foods, not to mention other good-for-you phytochemicals, hold the key.

Taking these substances as supplements doesn't have the same effect. For instance, research suggests eating vitamin C-rich foods could cut your risk of breast cancer and stomach cancer, but vitamin C supplements don't. You need the whole package that food gives you, perhaps because of the way phytochemicals and nutrients work together as a team.

This list gives you the names of some well-known phytochemicals, how experts think they boost health, and which foods are good sources. You can learn more about them by reading the related food chapters.

Phytochemicals

isothiocyanates (sulforaphane, others)	prevent cancer, partly by getting rid of cancer-causing compounds in your body	broccoli, brussels sprouts, cabbage, watercress, radish, horseradish, mustard
lignans (enterodiol, enterolactone, others)	help prevent ovarian and endometrial cancers, cardiovascular disease, and osteoporosis	flaxseed, sunflower seeds, legumes, whole grains, bran, berries, broccoli, cabbage, brussels sprouts
organosulfur compounds (allicin, others)	keep blood from clotting and improve cholesterol levels, may protect against colon and stomach cancers	garlic, onions, chives, shallots, leeks
indole-3-carbinol	prevents cancer by squashing free radicals, changing estrogen into a less cancer-causing form, and partly blocking estrogen's effect on cells	cruciferous veggies, like broccoli, brussels sprouts, cabbage, kale, cauliflower, collard greens, mustard greens

Carotenoids

carotenes (alpha and beta carotene)	reduce your risk of lung cancer and cardiovascular disease	spinach, carrots, sweet potatoes, kale, collards
xanthophylls (lutein, beta cryptoxanthin, zeaxanthin)	prevent cataracts and age-related macular degeneration	red peppers, papayas, oranges, spinach, kale
lycopene	protects against age-related macular degeneration, cataracts, cancer, and cardiovascular disease	tomatoes, pink grapefruit, guava, watermelon

Flavonoids (polyphenols)

anthocyanins	relieve arthritis and gout by blocking pain and inflammation, prevent plaque buildup in arteries	red, blue, and purple berries, red and purple grapes, red wine
flavonols (catechin, epicatechin, proanthocyanidins)	aid weight loss, protect against prostate cancer, slash heart disease risk, ward off type 2 diabetes, block urinary tract infections	green, black, oolong, and white teas, chocolate, apples, berries, red grapes, red wine
flavonols (resveratrol, quercetin, kaempferol, myricetin)	lower risk of lung and prostate cancers, keep cancer cells from multiplying and trigger them to die, dampen inflammation that leads to atherosclerosis	grape skins and seeds, wine, tea, yellow onions, scallions, kale, broccoli, apples, berries
isoflavones (genistein)	prevent breast and uterine cancer, guard against osteoporosis, ease menopausal hot flashes	soybeans, soy products, legumes

5 *Eat more fat –
the good kind*

"Fat" is not a bad word. Experts are starting to rethink recommen-dations to eat a low-fat diet, because some fats are actually good for your heart. Cooking with olive oil instead of butter, or eating fish instead of hamburger, is a tasty, easy, and painless way to watch your cholesterol, battle erratic heart rhythms (arrhythmias), prevent hardening of the arteries, and dodge heart disease.

Most foods contain a little fat, which is a good thing since you need some to function. A no-fat diet would ruin your health. Fats help you absorb important nutrients like vitamins A, D, E, and K. In fact, foods with these vital fat-soluble vitamins should be eaten with fat, so your body can absorb these crucial nutrients. Besides, fat makes foods flavorful, smooth, creamy, and more satisfying.

But not all fats are created equal. Some fats, like those rich in omega-3s, actually help prevent illness and obesity. Saturated and trans fats, which you'll read about later, harm your heart. Unsaturated fats, like these, protect it.

Monounsaturated fats (MUFAs). Foods that contain mostly MUFAs are liquid at room temperature — think olive or canola oil. This good fat triggers your body to make more HDL, or "good" cholesterol, while lowering both your total and "bad" LDL cholesterol. Avocados and nuts, including peanuts, are also great sources of MUFAs.

Polyunsaturated fats (PUFAs). These friendly fats come in two main types, both liquid at room temperature.

- Omega-6 may protect you from cardiovascular diseases such as heart attack, stroke, and heart disease by dropping your total and LDL cholesterol levels. Unfortunately, they may also lower your good HDL cholesterol. Corn, soybean, and safflower oils are packed with omega-6.

- Omega-3s help prevent arrhythmias and blood clots, plus lower your total cholesterol and triglycerides, all of which slash your risk of heart attack and heart-related death. Experts say you should try to eat at least one serving of an omega-3-rich food, like salmon, flaxseed, walnuts, or canola oil, every day.

Find a better balance

Ages ago, people used to eat about the same amount of omega-6 as omega-3. Now, you likely eat 10 times more omega-6 than omega-3, thanks to cooking with vegetable oil — high in omega-6 — and not eating enough omega-3-rich fish.

Even though these fats are good for you, you still need to limit your total fat (saturated, unsaturated, and trans fats) to 20 to 35 percent of your daily calories. Make sure most of that comes from polyunsaturated and monounsaturated fats. These ideas can help you get started.

- Ditch the butter and switch to olive oil. It's every bit as good for sautéing vegetables and stir-frying chicken, and it's a lot healthier.

- Make your own salad dressing with olive oil as a base and a dash of balsamic vinegar or lemon juice.

- Spruce up a plain salad with nuts, sunflower seeds, sliced avocado, and olives, all great sources of unsaturated fats.

- Grab a handful of peanuts instead of potato chips when you need a crunchy snack.

- Serve fish a few times each week. Fatty fish, such as salmon, are loaded with omega-3.

- Choose chicken over beef when you go grocery shopping. Chicken has many more PUFAs than beef, which may explain why eating chicken in place of red meat seems to lower your risk of heart disease.

- Cook with canola, corn, olive, safflower, soybean, cottonseed, or sunflower oil whenever you can in place of stick butter or margarine.

- Check the Nutrition Facts label on foods and buy those with fewer saturated and trans fats and more unsaturated fats.

Keep in mind that even good fats pack a whopping 9 calories per gram, more than twice the amount of carbohydrates or protein. Since your body stores extra calories as fat, boosting good fats without cutting back on bad fats can lead to weight gain, yet another risk factor for heart disease. So don't just eat more unsaturated fats. Use them to replace saturated and trans fats in your diet whenever possible.

6 *Trim saturated fat*

As good as some fats are for you, others are just as bad. Take saturated fat, for instance. It gives steak, bacon, and pork chops their savory flavor and milk and cheese their creaminess, but it also clogs your arteries.

Saturated fats boost the amount of cholesterol your liver makes, especially the amount of LDL, or "bad," cholesterol. In turn, having high total and LDL cholesterol raises your risk of heart disease, the number one killer in the United States.

Cutting back on saturated fat is one of the easiest, quickest ways to get a grip on cholesterol and protect yourself from heart disease. But your goal isn't to slash all fat from your diet. Simply replace some of the saturated fatty foods you eat, like beef, with foods that boast mostly unsaturated fat, like fish.

How big a difference will that make? Consider this. Say you currently get 15 percent of your daily calories from eating saturated fat. Replace 5 percent of that 15 with unsaturated fat, and experts say you'll drop your risk of heart attack or dying from heart disease an amazing 40 percent.

In real terms that means if you eat 2,000 calories a day and get 300 of those calories from saturated fat (15 percent), you would need to switch just 100 of those calories (5 percent) over to unsaturated fat. You'd still be eating the same amount of fat every day — only different kinds.

Experts say you should get no more than 7 percent of your daily calories from saturated fat, about 140 calories if you eat 2,000 calories a day. Fortunately, you can find easy ways to trim saturated fat and keep the taste of foods you love.

Rank your fats

Even saturated fat comes in shades of gray. The kind in butter and other dairy products gives the biggest boost to LDL cholesterol, followed by beef, and — least dangerous — cocoa and chocolate.

- Buy lean cuts of meat, like loin and round cuts.

- Trim away visible fat on meat and remove the skin from poultry before cooking.

- Choose reduced-, low-, or fat-free versions of dairy products whenever possible. You'll get the same amount of calcium but much less saturated fat.

- Try olive or canola oil in place of butter when stir-frying foods.

- Coat cookware with nonstick vegetable spray instead of butter, margarine, or shortening.

- Add butter to vegetables just before serving them rather than during cooking. You'll need less to get the same flavor.

- Oven-bake onion rings and french fries instead of frying them.

- Replace the butter in recipes with half butter and half oil.

- Try substituting applesauce, cottage cheese, or pureed bananas, prunes, or garbanzo beans for half the margarine or butter in baked goodies, such as cakes, muffins, brownies, and breads.

- Add a little sugar to cold, evaporated, fat-free milk and whip. Serve immediately in place of whipped cream topping, or use in place of heavy cream in recipes.

- Use low-fat yogurt instead of sour cream in dips, on baked potatoes, and in some cream sauces. Or try a half-and-half mixture of half low-fat yogurt and half sour cream. Low-fat yogurt can replace mayonnaise in cole slaw, too.

7 *Dodge trans fat*

If the boogeyman were a food, he'd probably be a trans fat. This type of fat is your heart's worst nightmare. It raises your bad LDL and total cholesterol levels, as well as your triglycerides, while lowering your good HDL cholesterol. Not even saturated fat does that. Plus, it makes your blood stickier and more likely to clot.

What's more, you're almost guaranteed a bigger belly if you keep eating foods loaded with trans fat. It adds more fat and moves fat you already have to your abdomen. Even if you eat only enough calories to maintain your weight, getting some of them as trans fat will actually cause you to gain weight and pack on belly fat. Obesity and high-fat diets are also linked to higher blood pressure. Eating trans fat can lead to insulin resistance, as well, boosting blood sugar and contributing to the development of type 2 diabetes.

Add it up and trans fat can send your heart disease risk through the roof, too. Some experts blame this dangerous fat for at least 30,000 heart disease deaths each year. In the respected Nurses' Health Study, women who ate the most trans fat — as little as 3 percent of their daily calories — had a 50-percent higher risk of heart disease than those who ate the least.

Maybe trans fats are more a case of Dr. Jekyll and Mr. Hyde. They start out good but, through some fancy chemistry, become very bad. They begin life as heart-healthy polyunsaturated fats, typically corn, soybean, safflower, sunflower, or cottonseed oil. When manufacturers add hydrogen to them, a process called hydrogenation, some of these PUFAs turn into saturated and trans fats.

But there's great news. Anyone — even seniors — can lower their blood pressure, blood sugar, and belly fat by cutting trans fat, and — therefore — total fat, in their diet. Start now, change just a few health habits, and live longer. These tips will help you spot trans fat and avoid it.

Read food labels. Don't rely on packages that promise "0 trans fat!" Foods can claim to be trans fat free as long as they have less than half a gram per serving. Unfortunately, a serving may be smaller than you think. Eat three or four in one sitting, and you can unwittingly eat a couple of grams of trans fat.

Instead, check the ingredient list on food labels for the words "partially hydrogenated vegetable oil" or "vegetable shortening" — telltale signs that a food contains man-made trans fat.

Buy better butter. Soft margarine in squeeze bottles and tubs packs less trans fat than stick margarine. But if you're really worried about your cholesterol, consider switching to a spread such as Benecol made with plant stanols, or Take Control made with plant sterols. These com-pounds help lower cholesterol. You can substitute Benecol in baking and cooking measure-for-measure in place of butter, margarine, shortening, or oil without changing the food's flavor.

Stick with liquids. Cook with oils such as canola, olive, corn, or other vegetable oils whenever you can rather than shortening, butter, or margarine. Why? Liquid fats, like oils, are mostly unsaturated, while solid fats are mostly saturated or trans.

Beware baked and fried foods. About 70 percent of the trans fat you eat probably comes from store-bought baked goods, like crackers, muffins, and cookies, and from fried foods served in fast food and other restaurants.

Get back to basics. Once research proved saturated fats were bad for your heart, scientists developed trans fats to replace them in food. Now scientists are scrambling to develop new fats to replace trans fats. Think twice before you buy in. Controversy surrounds the most promising replacements, called interesterified fats ("high stearate" or "stearic rich" oils on food labels). In one study, they sent after-meal blood sugar skyrocketing, while lowering HDL. Other studies say they're safe.

Your best bet is to eat more foods in their natural, fresh form and limit processed, prepackaged foods. Shop the produce section, skip the baked and fried goodies, and cook with healthy oils.

8 *Look for hidden salt*

Throughout history, salt has been used as a seasoning, a preservative, and even as money. Still, it plays a big part in your life, often because of the bad things it does to your body.

Salt contains both chloride and the mineral sodium. Your body needs a little sodium to live, but getting enough each day is not a problem. Getting too much is.

People ages 51 to 70 only need 1,300 milligrams (mg) of sodium a day, and adults over 70 need less, 1,200 mg. Although eating more than 2,300 mg of sodium a day isn't safe, an incredible 95 percent of men and 75 percent of women do just that.

Cutting back can help put a lid on high blood pressure and lower your risk for heart attack and stroke. And since chronic high blood pressure also damages your organs, especially kidneys, limiting sodium can also help prevent kidney disease. You'll fight back against osteoporosis, too, because a high-sodium diet makes you lose calcium through your urine. It also makes the bacterium *H. pylori,* the main cause of stomach and intestinal ulcers, more powerful. Lower your sodium and you drop your risk of stomach cancer and gastritis — inflammation of your stomach lining.

All in all, experts say healthy adults should cap sodium intake at 2,300 mg a day — the lower, the better. If you have high blood pressure, you need to aim for even less — no more than 1,500 mg a day.

Eat fewer processed foods. A whopping 75 percent of the salt you eat each day comes from prepackaged foods, not from the salt on your own table. Manufacturers add salt during processing to punch up flavor and lengthen a food's shelf life. Switch to eating more fresh fruits and vegetables, and you'll automatically eat less salt.

Read labels religiously. Breads and pastries that taste sweet, not salty, are actually some of the biggest contributors to dietary sodium. Read every food's label to avoid unpleasant surprises.

The Nutrition Facts panel tells you how many milligrams of sodium are in a single serving of food. Check the serving size against how much you plan to eat in one sitting. The ingredients list tells you whether the sodium comes from added salt or a preservative, like sodium benzoate.

Raid your medicine cabinet. Many over-the-counter and pre-scription drugs — from antacids and laxatives to pain relievers and cold medicines — contain sodium, too. Read package labels on OTCs and ask your pharmacist to check the inserts that come with prescription drugs.

Eat in, not out. Restaurants and fast food joints serve up huge portions of food and salt. The American Medical Association has called on the restaurant industry to cut its salt use in half over the next 10 years, but don't wait until then. Rein in your tendency to eat out, and cook with fresh ingredients at home.

Switch to a life-saving substitute. Consider swapping your regular salt for a potassium-enriched salt substitute made with half potassium chloride and half sodium chloride. You'll swing a one-two punch at heart disease by cutting sodium and boosting your potassium intake. New research shows using this seasoning could reduce deaths from heart disease, diabetes, high blood pressure, and stroke by 40 percent.

Potassium can be harmful in large amounts, especially if you have kidney disease or take certain medications, including ACE inhibitors and potassium-sparing diuretics such as spironolactone. Talk to your doctor before trying potassium salt substitutes if you fit this description.

Fend off foodborne illness

The Centers for Disease Control has unveiled the six most dangerous foods in the United States, and you might be surprised. One is a "health food," one a gourmet delicacy, and one might have been on your breakfast plate this morning. But you don't have to risk your health. Check this "most wanted" list to find tasty alternatives.

Unsafe food	Healthy substitute
raw fish (sushi)	baked, broiled, or poached salmon
alfalfa sprouts	washed romaine lettuce or spinach
raw oysters	steamed oysters
raw (unpasteurized) milk	pasteurized dairy products
runny eggs	eggs cooked until yolk is firm
undercooked hamburger and ground beef	ground beef cooked to an internal temperature of 160 degrees Fahrenheit

9 *Be picky about protein*

When you think of protein, maybe you imagine body builders and athletes. Yet, you need protein, too, and no other nutrient plays so many roles in your body. It helps build muscles, blood cells, scar tissue, hormones, hair, and nails — and more.

Proteins are long strands of tiny particles called amino acids. Each amino acid is like a letter of the alphabet, and proteins are the words they form when you put them together. Shuffle the letters around, and you create different proteins. Your body can make some amino acids. Others it can't, so you have to get them from food.

Luckily, a varied, balanced diet gives you all the amino acids, and protein, you need to thrive. Meat, fish, eggs, and dairy products usually provide complete protein — that means all the amino acids. Most plant foods, on the other hand, generally give you incomplete protein because they are missing a few amino acids.

Aside from the essential roles it plays in your body, adding lean protein to your breakfast can also help you lose weight without trying. In some amazing but true research, overweight women who started their day with a slice of Canadian bacon and American cheese on an English muffin felt fuller afterward and had less desire to munch. Experts think this early burst of protein could help you eat less during the rest of the day. In contrast, eating lots of protein throughout the day, every day did not blunt hunger.

That's important, because eating too much meat can have serious consequences. The problem for most meat eaters isn't getting enough protein — it's getting too much. Diets high in protein-rich foods are actually linked to obesity and can worsen existing kidney problems and increase calcium loss from your bones. Plus, focusing on foods with protein can crowd out other important nutrients, like vitamin C and folate. Plus, meat can come packaged with lots of saturated fat, calories, and cholesterol.

Balance is the key. You need protein to live, but not too much. Women only need around 50 grams of protein daily, while men need around 65 grams. You also need to be aware of where you get it.

Switch to fish. Eat fish instead of beef twice a week, and you'll not only get plenty of complete protein but also heart-protecting polyunsaturated omega-3 fats.

Lean toward legumes. One cup of cooked legumes, such as dry beans, peas, and lentils, provides about 30 percent of your daily protein. Plus, you reap the benefits of their rich stores of fiber and iron without the saturated fat and cholesterol you get with meat, whole milk, and other full-fat dairy products.

Cook with moist heat. It makes protein more digestible so you absorb more of it. Frying, on the other hand, makes it harder to digest.

Combine plant foods. Remember how amino acids are like alphabet letters, with most plant foods missing a few? Luckily, you can get all the letters by pairing up plant foods. Grains, for instance, give you one-half of the alphabet, while legumes give you the other. Eat them together and you get the whole alphabet of amino acids — complete protein. Beans with rice, peanut butter on bread, and tofu over brown rice are just a few such complementary combinations. You don't have to eat them together in the same meal, just in the same day.

10 *Drink more water*

Wars have been fought over water, and whole civilizations have been built around it, all because no one can live without it. In his book *Eat, Drink, and Be Healthy,* Harvard nutrition expert Walter Willett puts it this way — "You dry, you die."

Even minor dehydration can make you feel tired, grumpy, and constipated; cloud your concentration; and increase your risk of kidney stones and bladder cancer over time. Extreme dehydration can lead to heatstroke and death.

Your body is very good at conserving water, but you still need to replace what you lose through urine, breathing, and sweating. On average, scientists say people who eat 2,000 calories a day should drink eight 8-ounce glasses of fluids daily.

Not surprisingly, that number differs for everyone. The elderly often need more fluids, while people who eat lots of fruits and vegetables, which contain mostly water, may need less. You generally should drink more water during both the hottest and coldest times of year, when traveling on an airplane, when ill, if you're on a high-fiber diet, and on days when you're active. The best rule of thumb for normal days — drink at least one glass of water with each meal, and another in between meals.

Water does more than just keep you from dying, although that's one good reason to drink it. It adds to your life in other ways, too. Check out these fascinating facts.

- Drinking two glasses of water while sitting raises low blood pressure in people whose pressure normally drops when they stand up.

- On the other hand, drinking mineral-rich "hard" water could lower high blood pressure, heart disease risk, and your chances of dying from a heart attack. Fluoride in water seems to offer the most protection from heart disease, while iron and copper may raise your risk.

- Knowing what to drink can boost your energy. Fatigue is sometimes a symptom of heat exhaustion, not just a poor night's sleep. Water is the best beverage cure. And while caffeinated and sugary drinks may give you a temporary burst of energy, you'll crash a short while later. Turn to water for longer-lasting refreshment, along with other beverage favorites, like decaffeinated green, black, and herbal teas.

- Water that's suitable for drinking cleans cuts and scrapes just as well as saline solutions or distilled water.

- Washing your hands with plain tap water removes more of the dreaded norovirus, the leading cause of stomach flu, than washing with antibacterial soap or using an alcohol-based hand sanitizer. Water removed 96 percent of the virus, the antibacterial soap 88 percent, and hand gel a mere 46 percent in a recent study.

- Simply drinking four or more cups of water each day can help you lose an extra 2 pounds a year.

- Cutting all the sugary drinks from your diet and replacing them with water can help you lose an extra 5 pounds a year.

- Sipping ice-cold carbonated water can banish that sense of having something stuck in your throat, thus ending the cycle of continuous throat clearing.

None of this may matter if you can't stand the taste of your tap water. Treating public water with chlorine kills bacteria and viruses and makes it safe to drink, but it can leave an unpleasant flavor. Take the "ick" out of city water by chilling it in an uncovered pitcher before drinking, adding a splash of unsweetened fruit juice, or buying an inexpensive filter for your faucet or a Brita pitcher with a filter.

11 *Rediscover tea*

Asian people are some of the heaviest smokers in the world, yet they enjoy some of the lowest rates of cancer and heart disease. Scientists call this the "Asian paradox," but it may no longer be a mystery. Mounting evidence points to tea, Asia's main beverage, as the key.

Green, black, and oolong tea come from the same plant. Green tea is harvested from mature tea leaves, then steamed whole. The leaves for black tea are fermented first, which changes their chemical compounds. Oolong tea leaves are only partly fermented, so they boast some of the benefits of both (unfermented) green tea and (fermented) black tea.

All teas boast phytochemical compounds called flavonols. Green tea also contains catechins, another type of phytochemical with potent, disease-fighting powers. Fermenting the leaves forms new compounds, known as theaflavins and thearubigins. Green tea has more catechins than black tea, but black tea is rich in theaflavins and thearubigins. Oolong tea contains all three compounds.

Tea offers serious defense against cavities, in part because the leaves naturally contain fluoride. In addition, lab studies show green, black, and oolong tea extracts keep cavity-causing bacteria from growing and producing acid that eats away tooth enamel. Beware of instant tea. Some brands contain more fluoride than the Environmental Protection Agency and Food and Drug Administration deem safe.

Green tea. This powerful beverage packs more antioxidants than either black or oolong tea. In lab studies, it shows promise for preventing cancer of the colon, breast, stomach, lung, pancreas, esophagus, and bladder. It also seems to slow the spread of prostate cancer when used alongside a class of drugs called COX-2 inhibitors.

Need more reasons to try it? Drinking at least two cups a day may cut your risk of skin cancer by protecting you from ultraviolet (UV) rays. Plus, green tea may help prevent high blood pressure, lower blood sugar, soothe arthritis inflammation, and block bladder inflammation. And in one recent study, Japanese adults who drank six or more cups a day were less likely to develop type 2 diabetes.

Just like the rest of your body, there are foods that'll keep your brain razor sharp. For instance, lab studies in mice suggest a couple of cups a day of green tea could do a lot to help keep your mind young. Scientists think catechins, the antioxidants in green tea, may protect brain cells from oxidative damage that accumulates with age. This, in turn, could help preserve your memory and learning ability well into old age.

Green tea is safe as a beverage, but supplements may harm your liver. Drinking huge amounts of green tea — half a gallon or more each day — may make the drug warfarin (Coumadin) less effective.

Black tea. If you can't get rid of stress, at least drink a cup of black tea. Evidence suggests getting comfortable with a "cuppa" fights damaging stress hormones. Two cups a day could lower your risk of ovarian cancer by 30 percent and reduce colon cancer risk. What's more, black tea seems to slash your risk for cardiovascular disease. Heart attack protection begins at just three cups a day, while four to five cups daily fights heart disease by relaxing your arteries.

You can even drink it to boost your bones and battle osteoporosis. Numerous studies show black tea increases bone density and protects against hip fractures, especially if you drink four or more cups a day. Adding milk will bump up your calcium intake, too, and further guard your bones.

Oolong tea. This drink with the funny name makes a big impression. It seems to promote weight loss and lower triglycerides, and research links it to lower blood sugar in people with type 2 diabetes. Like other teas, it, too, boasts cancer-preventing compounds — namely caffeine, theaflavins, and thearubigins.

Still, too much of a good thing can be bad. Drinking more than three quarts a day of oolong or black tea can lead to hypokalemia, a potentially deadly condition linked to caffeine toxicity.

Tea time tips

Enjoy a little milk with your tea. Experts once thought milk neutralized the antioxidants in tea, but new research proves otherwise. So have a dash of milk with your "cuppa."

The natural flavonoids in black, green, and oolong teas, however, can keep your body from absorbing iron in food. Sidestep this side effect by drinking water, not tea, with meals.

---

12 *Make peace with coffee*

Coffee has had a conflicted history, with the legends surrounding it dating as far back as the third century. Early monks loved it because it helped them stay awake during long evening prayers. In the 17th century, some devout Catholics declared coffee sinful. Pope Clement saved the day by baptizing the brew, cementing its approval by the church. Undoubtedly, sleepy monks everywhere rejoiced.

Coffee was on the outs again until recently. Early research linked this brew to breast cancer, pancreatic cancer, and heart disease. But these studies didn't take into account the fact that many coffee drinkers also smoked — the real villain behind these deadly diseases. Scientists these days are seeing the light and singing the praises, or at least the safety, of coffee consumed in moderation.

Caffeine gets the most attention, but coffee contains more than 1,000 compounds, most of which affect your health. It packs more soluble fiber, the kind that dissolves in water, than orange juice and is a major source of antioxidants, including chlorogenic acid. Based on recent research, that could add up to:

- a lower type 2 diabetes risk for drinking decaf, and an even lower risk for drinking regular coffee. Experts say you may need to drink more than four cups daily to reap this benefit, which might not be safe for some people.

- lower risk of death from heart disease in people over the age of 65 who don't have severely high blood pressure.

- 40 percent less chance of developing Parkinson's disease, at least in men.

- protection from liver disease, as well as colon, rectal, and liver cancers.

- fewer gout attacks since coffee seems to lower uric acid levels.

- less mental decline with age in people who drink three or more cups of coffee daily.

- lower risk of getting gallstones and kidney stones.

Keep in mind, coffee — particularly the caffeinated kind — can have unpleasant side effects if you drink too much — jitteriness, irritability, and insomnia, to name a few. Drinking coffee that doesn't go through a paper filter, like espresso and French press, can also raise your cholesterol a few points. Maybe more worrisome, drinking a lot of coffee, roughly four or more cups a day, may speed up bone loss and put you at higher risk for hip fracture. Experts say keeping your coffee habit to three or fewer cups a day should be safe.

Skip this to sleep better

Having trouble sleeping through the night? Caffeine may not be the culprit. Instead, try cutting down on alcohol in the evening. A hot toddy may help you unwind at first, but alcohol actually disrupts your brain waves, making it harder to fall asleep and stay asleep.

People with diabetes shouldn't start drinking joe if they don't already, since caffeine can temporarily raise blood sugar. Evidence links coffee to higher blood pressure, too, so you may want to avoid it if you already face a higher risk for heart problems.

13 *Add variety to meals*

If all the hype over what to eat and what not to eat makes you want to give up your good intentions and grab a bag of chips, just remember this simple rule — eat a variety of food every day.

The most important food you can eat for more energy, a more youthful body, and a longer life is any healthy food you enjoy and didn't eat already today. The U.S. Department of Agriculture, which provides the Food Pyramid and other guidelines, offers these tips.

- Enjoy something from each food group every day — vegetables; fruits; grains; dairy; and meat, beans, and nuts.

- Eat each type of veggie several times a week — dark green vegetables (broccoli, spinach), orange vegetables (carrots, sweet potatoes), legumes (dry beans, chickpeas), starchy vegetables (corn, peas, white potatoes), and other vegetables (tomatoes, cauliflower, celery).

- Limit the amount of saturated and trans fats, cholesterol, alcohol, added sugar, and salt you consume.

Why the emphasis on eating a little of everything? Each food group is the main source of at least one nutrient. No food group provides all the nutrients you need. That means falling short on one or more types of food also shortchanges your body of nutrients. What's more, no single nutrient can stand alone. They work together in your body, so a deficiency in one affects all the others.

While you're adding variety to your meals, aim for nutrition density, too. Nutrient-dense foods are those that pack a lot of vitamins, minerals, phytochemicals, and other good-for-you compounds but relatively few calories. Think fresh strawberries and peaches, steamed asparagus and broccoli, or a delicious salmon steak. Now hold the butter, cream sauce, and extra sugar, and you have a nutrient-dense meal.

Focusing on nutritious, low-calorie foods with little added sugar will give you all the nutrients you need to stay healthy and allow you to enjoy occasional treats, without gaining weight. Best of all, you won't feel like you are depriving yourself.

14 Get a handle on food labels

You've seen the ingredients list and nutrition information on food packages. Maybe you've even read them. But what good are food labels, really? For starters, they can point you to healthier food choices, plus help you maintain a healthy weight, protect your heart, beat high blood sugar, and avoid allergic reactions to food.

Tally the numbers. Before you put that package in your grocery cart, check the Nutrition Facts panel for this basic information.

- *Serving size.* This is a standard amount set by the government so you can compare similar foods. It's not usually a recommended amount. Pay close attention to the serving size. It may be smaller than what you actually eat, so you may be getting more calories, fat, and sugar than the label suggests.

- *Calories.* The total amount of energy you get from eating one serving. Keeping an eye on this number and choosing foods with fewer calories can help you slim down, which in turn cuts your risk for obesity-related illnesses, like type 2 diabetes.

- *Fats.* This includes total fat in a single serving, as well as the different types of fat and the amount of each. In general, pick foods with the least amount of trans and saturated fats, and more monounsaturated or polyunsaturated fats.

- *Daily Value (DV).* How much of your daily allotment of fiber, fat, vitamins, minerals, and other nutrients you get from each serving. Unfortunately, DVs don't take into account your gender, age, or activity level. They are based on eating 2,000 calories each day, which may be too many or too few for you. Use them as a general nutritional guide.

Eye added ingredients. The ingredients list tells you everything in a food, from most to least, and helps you spot unhealthy extras. Avoid foods that list added sugar, hydrogenated oil, sodium, or another unhealthy ingredient among the first three in the list — a sure sign the food contains a lot of it. Added sugar, in particular, parades under sneaky names, including sucrose, dextrose, maltose, corn syrup, high-fructose corn syrup, and fruit juice concentrate. And if the food contains added MSG, aspartame, or sulfites, you'll find them listed here.

Ferret out food allergens. The Food and Drug Administration (FDA) now requires labels to tell you in clear language if the food is made with milk, eggs, wheat, fish, soybeans, peanuts, tree nuts — like almonds, walnuts, and pecans — or shellfish, such as shrimp or lobster. Don't take a chance if you're allergic to these ingredients. Even foods like nondairy creamer may contain milk protein. Check the ingredients list for these allergens or look for the word "Contains," as in "Contains soy, wheat, and milk."

Get wise to health claims. Splashy ads like "Fat free" and "No sugar added" can help you make healthier decisions about what goes in your buggy. But you can't rely on these claims alone. Some healthy foods that are allowed to make these claims don't. What's more, these statements can be misleading. Manufacturers can make a food sound healthier than it really is through clever advertising. For instance, a "fat free" food can have just as many calories as the full-fat version if it makes up for lost taste with loads of sugar.

It pays to compare the Nutrition Facts panel and ingredients list of different brands. On the following page, you'll find a chart of some commonly used claims and what they really mean. All numbers are per serving.

Claim	What it means
calorie free	less than five calories
low calorie	no more than 40 calories
reduced calorie	at least 25 percent fewer calories than the regular version
good source of calcium	at least 100 milligrams (mg) of calcium
good source of (any nutrient)	10 to 19 percent of the recommended daily value (DV) for that nutrient
high in, rich in, or excellent source of (any nutrient)	20 percent or more of the DV for that nutrient
light or lite	one-third fewer calories or half the fat of the regular version or half the sodium of a low-calorie, low-fat food; may also refer to the texture or color of the product, as in "light brown sugar"

15 *Take control of portions*

Size matters. Plopping a large portion of food on your plate can actually prompt you to overeat, because most people will eat until their plate is clean. When supersize portions become the norm, as they have at fast food and other restaurants, you can say goodbye to your waistline and hello to a higher risk for obesity-related illnesses.

The answer to living longer and living better isn't necessarily a special no-fat, no-carb, or vegetarian diet. It's much simpler than that.

New research shows eating a low-calorie diet can extend your life, improve how you feel every day, and maybe even prevent or slow the progress of Alzheimer's. Trimming calories can also help you lose weight, which in turn can lower high blood pressure.

Luckily, you can painlessly fool yourself into eating less and feel full, not deprived. Begin with these 10 best healthy eating tips for losing weight permanently and lowering your blood pressure quickly and naturally.

- Only use tall, skinny glasses to hold high-calorie beverages, like soft drinks and alcohol. People tend to pour about 30 percent more liquid when using short, wide glasses.

- Serve your meals on smaller plates, in smaller bowls, and with smaller spoons, and you'll automatically eat less. Large plates make a normal-size portion look small, while small plates make it look larger. And hide the supersized serving ware. Serve yourself with a large spoon, and you'll scoop up extra-large portions.

- Plump up your food to make it look bigger, and your tummy won't notice you're really eating less. Whip air into foods to make them thick and creamy, and add lots of lettuce, tomato, and other low-calorie condiments to small burger patties.

- Compare portions to common objects. A cup of pasta is the size of a tennis ball, 3 ounces of fish is the size of a checkbook, and 3 ounces of meat a deck of cards. A teaspoon of butter or margarine is the size of a die, while two tablespoons of salad dressing fill one shot glass.

- Make getting seconds more of a hassle. Leave serving dishes in the kitchen or on a sideboard at least 6 feet away from where you eat. As the saying goes, out of sight, out of mind.

- Don't clear away empty platters, dirty dishes, or leftover bones from the dinner table right away. Leaving the remnants helps you remember how much you have eaten and makes you less likely to overeat.

- Watch what you eat when dining with others. Research shows people eat 35 percent more when dining with one other person than when eating alone, and 96 percent more when dining with a group of seven or more people.

- Never snack straight from the package. Put your snack on a clean plate and sit down at the table to eat. Don't stand in the kitchen or watch TV while snacking.

- Buy prepackaged, 100-calorie snacks or save money by divvy-ing up your own single-serving portions into sandwich bags. When you crave a bite, grab a ready-made bag to keep yourself from overeating.

- Beware of indulging in "low-fat" foods. They only have about 15 percent fewer calories than their full-fat counterparts, yet studies show people eat up to 50 percent more of them in one sitting, just because they're labeled low fat.

All-you-can-eat foods

You can eat virtually as much as you want of some foods. Most fruits and vegetables, broth-based soups, and skim milk fall into this category. They contain lots of water, loads of nutrients, and few calories. All that volume can also fill you up and keep you full longer.

In fact, research shows starting each meal with a bowl of broth-based soup will actually help you lose weight — even if you're adding an extra course. As an appetizer, it will fill you up and help you eat less of your entrée. So sip yourself slim. Just be sure not to add calories to your main meal with toppings like butter or extra sugar.

16 *Cook it right*

How you cook your meals has almost as much to do with how healthy they are as what you cook. Vegetables retain more nutrients if cooked lightly with a minimum amount of water, for instance. The way you cook meat determines the amount of cancer-causing compounds, or carcinogens, it contains. Here's an easy-to-follow guide for preparing delicious, nutritious meals.

Steaming. Steam vegetables over water whenever possible. This method retains the most nutrients, plus plenty of flavor, crispness, and color — as long as you don't overcook your food.

Boiling. Minerals and some vitamins dissolve in water, so boiling can leach many good-for-you nutrients out of food and into the water. Pour that water down the drain, and you've lost up to half the nutrients in your food.

If you decide to boil certain vegetables, like potatoes, scrub them in water with a soft brush. Avoid soaking them. Add to boiling, not cold, water to minimize the time they spend in liquid, and don't cook them longer than necessary. Use the leftover "pot liquor" to moisten cornbread or add to soups and gravies.

Stir-frying. Cooking foods over high heat for a short amount of time in a little oil, like peanut oil, actually helps conserve their nutrients. For added iron in your food, consider stir-frying in a cast iron skillet. Then again, the iron will destroy vitamin C in your vegetables, so decide which nutrient you need most.

Microwaving. "Nuking" french fries before frying them helps reduce the formation of carcinogens because the fries spend less time in the hot oil. Most nutrition experts believe microwaving vegetables generally does not destroy their nutrients, as long as you use little or no water. However, microwaving cruciferous vegetables, like broccoli, cauliflower, and cabbage, on high power may destroy more nutrients, especially those helpful phytochemicals, than steaming.

Grilling. It's a summer staple, but grilling creates carcinogens such as heterocyclic amines (HCAs). In general, the longer you cook the meat and the higher the heat, the more HCAs form. Out of all cooking methods, grilling produces the most, followed by pan-frying and broiling. Poaching, stewing, baking, and stir-frying produce the least. Luckily, disarming these deadly compounds is simple.

- A day or two before you grill out, eat lots of cruciferous vegetables, such as broccoli, cauliflower, kale, cabbage, and brussels sprouts. They're chock full of anti-cancer compounds that help neutralize HCAs in your body.

- Marinate chicken, ribs, and other meats for 40 minutes in a mixture of olive oil, brown sugar, cider vinegar, garlic, mustard, lemon juice, and salt.

- Partially cook meat, including hamburger patties, in the microwave for a few minutes before throwing it on the grill. Dump out the juices that accumulate on the cooking dish.

- Flip your burgers once a minute while grilling. This prevents up to 100 percent of HCAs, most likely by keeping meat from getting too hot.

- Don't serve meat "well done." Only cook until the meat thermometer reads between 165 and 180 degrees for poultry; 160 to 170 degrees for pork, lamb, and ground beef; and 145 to 160 degrees for roasts and beef steaks.

17 *Spice it up*

By using them in place of salt, spices can help you avoid high blood pressure and add delicious flavor to your meals. And as a bonus, many are rich in antioxidants. See how these three popular seasonings stack up.

Cinnamon. This spice can help stop diabetes in its tracks. Plus, it tastes great and is probably in your pantry right now. Compounds in cinnamon seem to act like insulin in your body, helping move sugar from your bloodstream into cells. As a result, it shows promise in preventing insulin resistance, which can lead to type 2 diabetes, and dampening after-meal blood sugar spikes in people who already have this disease.

Try sprinkling ground cinnamon onto cereal, oatmeal, yogurt, and toast, or add it to a hot cup of tea. Monitor your blood sugar closely to avoid hypoglycemia or low blood sugar, and don't make the mistake of eating cinnamon oil — it's toxic even in small amounts.

Cinnamon may also drop total cholesterol levels up to 26 percent and LDL cholesterol 27 percent. Research suggests as little as one-half teaspoon daily is all it takes to lower triglycerides as much as 30 percent. Finally, recent studies have shown this common spice has the ability to block inflammation. Experts think inflammation plays a role in many diseases, particularly those associated with growing older. So cinnamon may help you ward off the big three of aging — arthritis, heart disease, and Alzheimer's.

Ginger. Research proves ginger relieves the nausea and vomiting that sometimes strike after surgery and may treat motion and seasickness, as well. And unlike anti-nausea drugs, this natural cure won't make you drowsy.

It could even ease the pain of osteoarthritis and rheumatoid arthritis, according to some studies. What's more, lab research shows this super root kills cancer cells, while others suggest it improves insulin sensitivity in diseases like diabetes.

For these benefits, try getting two teaspoons of fresh, grated ginger twice a day. Or, to make a zinging tea, grate three teaspoons of fresh ginger, add to one cup of cold water, and bring to a boil in a tightly covered, non-aluminum pan. Simmer for 10 minutes over low heat, then remove and let stand covered for five minutes. Drink while it's hot.

Ginger has a long history of being safe. However, it can cause heartburn, diarrhea, and mouth irritation in some people, and increase your risk of bleeding if you take blood-thinning drugs, such as warfarin (Coumadin).

Mustard. Cooking with this common spice may ease many respiratory problems, such as chest congestion, bronchitis, bronchial cough, and sinusitis.

Herbal healers suggest making a paste from powdered black mustard seeds and warm water, wrapping it in linen, and laying it across your chest for 10 to 15 minutes to relieve congestion. Mustard can irritate your skin, however, so think twice before trying this folk remedy. Rubbing olive oil onto your skin after removing the paste may ease the irritation.

18 *Feel good about snacking*

Snacking can be a healthy habit, if you do it right. Make nutritious choices and munch in moderation, and you are on your way to filling your belly and lengthening your life. Try these tips to get started.

Follow the 5/20 rule. Use the Nutrition Facts panel on packages to choose food with less than 5 percent of the Daily Value (DV) of saturated fat, trans fat, sodium, and sugar and more than 20 percent DV of fiber and individual vitamins and minerals.

Indulge in dark chocolate. Enjoy a few pieces of dark chocolate in place of your usual snack of cookies or crackers. Aside from being a decadent treat, dark chocolate is packed with phytochemicals called polyphenols that may widen arteries, lower blood pressure, and prevent blood clots. It may also boost blood flow to the brain, counteracting the effects of tiredness and aging on brain function. Milk chocolate doesn't have the same benefits.

Consider hot chocolate made with real cocoa and low-fat milk as an alternative to tea and wine. A cup of hot cocoa has nearly twice the antioxidants of red wine, three times more than green tea, and five times more than black tea. Experts say ounce for ounce, drinking cocoa is better than eating chocolate bars because it contains much less saturated fat.

Eat smaller meals more often. New research links eating six or more mini-meals a day with having a better cholesterol profile. This strategy may also keep you from feeling the urge to eat too much.

Cut back on sugary snacks. Canadian researchers discovered people with higher "good" HDL cholesterol tend to eat fewer servings of sodas, sweetened fruit juices, and sugary foods. If you tend to crave sweets, scientists say you may find it easier to snack on fruit than vegetables.

Fight fatigue with apricots

They may just be the perfect snack. Packed with iron, they help battle anemia. Plus, they're an excellent source of beta carotene, an antioxidant your body turns into vitamin A. This nutrient combats hypothyroidism by helping your thyroid absorb iodine. Add to that their natural sugar, and you get a quick, midday pick-me-up. Dried apricots are particularly potent because their nutrients are more concentrated, making them a healthy — and handy — on-the-go snack.

Find comfort in new foods. Comfort foods aren't known for being healthy, but they can be. A bowl of sherbet or low-fat frozen yogurt can feel just as comforting as a bowl of full-fat, cookie-dough ice cream.

Make favorites more wholesome. Instead of buying buttered popcorn, pop the plain or low-fat variety and sprinkle on fat-free butter-flavored sprinkles, cheese flavoring, or salt. Like chips? Crunch on corn and tortilla chips fried in corn, canola, or sunflower oils, all rich in healthy polyunsaturated fats. New research shows eating these chips in place of other high-fat snacks can lower your triglycerides along with total and LDL cholesterol.

Don't deprive yourself. Instead of cutting certain foods completely from your diet, simply eat them in smaller portions or as an occasional reward. By bagging a few cookies in sandwich bags beforehand, you can satisfy sweet-tooth attacks without going overboard.

Chew gum to resist cravings. In a new study, men and women who chewed gum after a meal dampened their cravings for an in-between snack, especially a sweet snack, compared to those who didn't chew gum.

Limit distractions. It's so tempting to munch mindlessly while watching television or reading the newspaper. But studies find you are more likely to overeat when you are distracted. Put snacks on a plate and eat them at the table, and never nibble straight from the package.

Travel light. Wolfing fatty, sugary foods on the go can lead to overeating and grogginess behind the wheel. If you must eat in the car, plan ahead and prepare nutritious snacks to take with you, such as baby carrots, raisins, or a fresh plum.

19 *Dine defensively*

Eating fast food regularly can cause weight gain and insulin resistance. Those are the findings from a study funded by the National Institutes of Health (NIH). Both men and women, black and white, who ate fast food regularly over the course of 15 years gained an average of nearly 10 pounds and became twice as likely to develop insulin resistance, two major risk factors for type 2 diabetes.

That's probably no surprise, given the amount of fat and sugar in most restaurant food. Dining out doesn't have to be unhealthy. You can enjoy an occasional meal out and still be kind to your body.

Minimize, don't supersize. You can't control all the ingredients in restaurant food, but you can control how much you eat. The researchers behind the NIH study blame the bad results, in part, on enormous portions.

When grabbing fast food on the go, order the child-size portions, like the junior burger, or a half sandwich instead of a whole. Never get a double- or triple-patty burger. In sit-down restaurants, order the appetizer as your entrée, or split an entrée with a friend. You'll eat less and save money.

Spot better selections. Look for chicken and fish that have been grilled, broiled, or baked, not breaded or fried. And hold the fatty toppings. A baked potato makes for healthy fast food fare, but not if you top it with butter, sour cream, cheese, and bacon bits. Instead, order a small bowl of plain chili to pour on top. In restaurants, ask for rice steamed rather than fried, and order tacos and burritos topped with salsa in place of sour cream and cheese.

Avoid not-so-healthy salads. Just because you find macaroni salad at the salad bar does not mean it's good for you. Taco salads seated in a deep fried tortilla shell or topped with fried tortilla chips aren't any better. Skip salads with breaded or fried chicken and shrimp, and hold the extras — like bacon, croutons, and cheese. Order dressing on the side and only use half of it.

Get special treatment. Request low-fat or fat-free versions of salad dressing, mayonnaise, sour cream, cheese, and milk. Ask for spicy mustard instead of regular on sandwiches to make up for the lost flavor of high-fat dressings. Order a veggie pizza with half the regular cheese and sprinkle on your own Parmesan cheese and seasonings. And if you aren't sure how much sodium, saturated, or trans fat a food contains, ask.

Drink to good health. Water comes in number one for health, since it has no sugar, fat, or calories. Unsweetened tea and diet soda are runners-up. You can treat yourself with an occasional sweet tea, regular soda, or milkshake, but don't make them a habit. They're loaded with calories and sugar, and shakes are chock-full of fat.

20 Consider taking a multivitamin

No solid evidence proves taking a multivitamin-mineral supplement will help you dodge disease, but no study proves it will hurt you, either. Experts say it's usually a matter of choice. Most people don't need a nutritional supplement if they eat a well-balanced diet full of fruits, vegetables, beans, and whole grains. However, if you are on a strict diet or don't have the appetite you once did, you may want to take a multi-vitamin-mineral supplement. Here's how you can reap the benefits.

Supplement warning

Loading up on foods rich in beta carotene, like carrots, is good for you. Loading up on beta carotene supplements may not be. Research shows the supplements make smokers and people exposed to asbestos more likely to develop lung cancer, and they won't protect you from heart disease, diabetes, cataracts, or other types of cancer.

■ Check the label and look for a supplement that gives you no more than 100 percent of your daily nutrients. More than that can endanger your health.

■ Consider supplements made just for seniors. They're usually low in iron and vitamin A, which most older adults need little of, and rich in calcium and vitamins B6 and B12, which you generally need more of with age.

■ Don't buy a supplement that gives you more than 5,000 International Units (IU) of vitamin A daily. At least 20 percent of the vitamin A should be in the form of beta carotene.

■ Take vitamins and minerals with food to boost their absorption, unless the directions say otherwise.

If you opt out of taking a multivitamin-mineral supplement, talk to your doctor about getting these nutrients as stand-alone supplements.

Say yes to calcium and vitamin D. These two nutrients work together to shore up bone density. In combination, they help prevent osteoporosis and lower your risk of fractures, although calcium supplements can increase your chance of kidney stones. Research suggests you need 700 to 800 IU of vitamin D, along with 1,000 milligrams of calcium daily to reap these benefits.

Check out other supplements. Other vitamins and minerals show promise in preventing serious illnesses, like cancer and heart disease, but studies aren't conclusive. Discuss the pros and cons with your doctor before taking them.

- Selenium. Taking 200 micrograms (mcg) a day may help prevent lung, colon, prostate, and liver cancer.

- Vitamin E. Overall, it may prevent prostate and colon cancer in men who smoke, as well as protect women over age 65 from sudden, heart-related death. Vitamin E supplements may make nosebleeds more common, but they do not seem to increase your risk of serious bleeding, such as hemorrhagic stroke.

Information is your best protection against harmful reactions between supplements and medications. Before you use an herbal or nutritional supplement, you can make sure it's safe by checking the government's Web site *http://MedlinePlus.gov*. Click on "Drugs and Supplements" to look them up alphabetically and learn about dangerous interactions and proven benefits. Don't combine nutritional supplements with your medication without talking with your doctor or pharmacist first. The results could be deadly.

Top 10 powerhouse foods

These super foods give you fiber, vitamins, minerals, antioxidants, and more. Plus, they're low in calories and are readily available. Take the first step toward a healthy diet by eating the foods on this important list.

salmon	wheat bran
oatmeal	cabbage
flaxseeds	garlic
blueberries	pomegranates
black beans	green tea

Score big with vitamin-packed veggies

Artichokes

■ ■ ■ ■ ■ ■ ■ ■ ■ ■ ■ ■ ■ ■ ■ ■ ■

Ancient veggie bursts with nutrients

According to legend, the Ancient Romans adored French or globe artichokes and ate them with vinegar, honey, and cumin. Although this artichoke nearly vanished when the Roman Empire fell, it was still grown in Sicily and Spain. But in the 1500s, Catherine de Medici introduced artichokes to France when she married the French king. They've been popular ever since.

The artichoke is actually a green flower bud from a plant called *Cynara scolymus.* You can eat the outer leaves once you remove the tough tips, but don't eat the core "choke" or pale inner leaves. Instead try the firm, edible bottom beneath the choke that is usually called the artichoke heart. Real artichoke hearts or "baby artichokes" are tiny whole artichokes that have little or no choke.

Artichokes are low in saturated fat and cholesterol. They're also a good source of nutrients that help your body fight off disease.

Battle the brittle bones of osteoporosis. Calcium and vitamin D are the two nutrients you need most to keep your bones strong. But they need help, and surprisingly, artichokes are full of vitamins and minerals that fight bone loss.

- *Vitamin K.* A lack of this important vitamin will contribute to weaker bones, which could easily lead to a

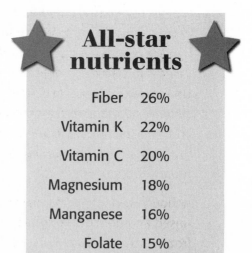

All-star nutrients

Nutrient	Daily Value
Fiber	26%
Vitamin K	22%
Vitamin C	20%
Magnesium	18%
Manganese	16%
Folate	15%

Serving size is 1 medium
Percent is Daily Value

fracture. But eating a medium artichoke can give you around a fifth of the daily vitamin K you need. Be careful though — vitamin K is a blood thinner so if you take warfarin or another blood-thinning medicine, you need to talk to your doctor before adding more to your diet.

- *Magnesium.* Sixty percent of your body's magnesium is in your skeleton, and some studies say low magnesium levels could be one of the causes of thinning bones. Fortunately, eating artichokes can add magnesium back into your diet.

- *Vitamin C.* Like magnesium, collagen is a crucial ingredient for strong bones. Your body can make its own collagen as long as you get enough vitamin C. A medium artichoke delivers 20 percent of your daily requirement. Dip the leaves in scrumptious salsa to add a bit more of this bone-saving nutrient.

Artichokes also contain manganese and copper. These trace minerals also play a role in building your bones and will help you win your war against osteoporosis.

■ ■ ■ ■ ■ Boost the benefits ■ ■ ■ ■ ■

Pre-packaged artichoke hearts can save extra work, because the cleaning and cutting is done for you — but be careful which kind you choose. Marinated artichoke hearts are packed in delicious olive oil and vinegar. Unfortunately, those extra ingredients add plenty of calories, so marinated artichoke hearts are a less healthy choice. You could try canned artichoke hearts instead, but they are usually packed in brine and may contain more salt than you need.

Although canned or marinated artichoke hearts can be rinsed and drained, your best and speediest bet may be frozen artichoke hearts. These have no oil or salt added, so they give you the most nutrition for the least effort.

Cut your risk of stroke. Artichokes may not look like stroke fighters, but they supply four power-hitter nutrients that can help you avoid this serious condition.

- *Vitamin C.* One of the surprising things about artichokes is they're a good source of vitamin C. A 10-year research study from Finland found that people who got the least vitamin C had a higher stroke risk, especially those who were overweight and had high blood pressure. If you think you may be low in this vital nutrient, adding artichokes to your diet can help.

- *Fiber.* If you have high blood pressure or high cholesterol, you're at higher risk for stroke. Fortunately, artichokes are loaded with stroke-fighting fiber. One artichoke will give you more than a quarter of your daily requirement. This fiber not only sweeps some cholesterol out of your body, it also lowers blood pressure.

- *Folate.* Researchers have long known that folate can help lower high levels of homocysteine in your blood. That helps prevent the blood clots that block blood flow to your brain, causing an ischemic stroke. But now Swedish research suggests folate also may help prevent hemorrhagic stroke, which is caused by a burst blood vessel.

- *Magnesium.* About one out of every six strokes results from a heart problem called atrial fibrillation, a clot-causing vibration in the upper chambers of your heart. If your body lacks magnesium, your risk of atrial fibrillation increases. Fortunately, one delectable medium artichoke delivers nearly a fifth of the magnesium you need each day.

Defend your lungs from asthma. A new study shows that two nutrients found in artichokes might lower your risk of asthma. People in the study who ate less vitamin C and manganese were more likely to have asthma symptoms. As a result, researchers think the antioxidant powers of vitamin C and manganese may help protect your lungs against this serious breathing condition. Because a medium artichoke can deliver at least 15 percent of the vitamin C and manganese you need each day, it's a good place to start. But don't stop there. Researchers also recommend getting vitamin C and manganese from fresh fruits such as pineapple.

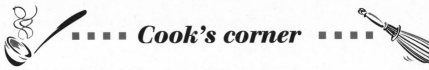

Cook's corner

- Before you buy a whole artichoke, squeeze it so the leaves press together. It will squeak when fresh. Bypass any artichoke that is opening into full bloom, drying out, woody, wilting, or has mold.

- If you can't eat artichokes the day you buy them, don't wash or trim them. Instead, drop them in a sealed plastic bag with a damp paper towel. Store in the fridge for up to a five days.

- Before you cook a whole artichoke, cut off the inch of leaf tips along the top and any other sharp leaf ends. Cut off the stem and remove any short leaves to make the bottom flat. Now it can stand on end when you cook it.

- To prevent a trimmed artichoke from turning brown, dip it in lemon juice.

- To eat the tasty artichoke leaves from a whole artichoke, pull off a leaf, dip it into a low-fat sauce like salsa, and pull the leaf through your teeth to remove the yummy part. Throw out that leaf before grabbing the next one.

Asparagus
■ ■ ■ ■ ■ ■ ■ ■ ■ ■ ■ ■ ■ ■ ■ ■ ■

Unique vegetable a food to be prized

Asparagus spears may have the bold look of plants from the primeval wilds, but asparagus comes from the same plant family as flowering lily-of-the-valley. You may be surprised to learn that this unique vegetable has been a luxury food for centuries.

Today, it's still a food to be prized. Before you select your velvety-tipped spears at the supermarket, they spend at least two seasons in the field. Then they must be picked by hand and shipped in a special container to preserve freshness. All this effort helps preserve many fragile but powerful nutrients, including a variety of vitamins, minerals, and phytonutrients. Yet this classy veggie has almost no cholesterol or fat. But one word of caution. Asparagus is the top source of the amino acid asparagine and has a high water content, so it may act as a diuretic.

Benefit from four cancer fighters in one spear. Make asparagus the spearhead in your cancer defense, and your digestive system might thank you. That's because four key nutrients in asparagus are already showing their cancer-fighting promise in research studies.

Vitamin A. A new study from Sweden shows that nonsmokers who ate the most vitamin A — as well as beta carotene and alpha carotene, which turn into vitamin A — were much less likely to develop stomach cancer. A few asparagus spears give you a good start on beta carotene. To add alpha carotene, add a side of carrots or a piece of pumpkin pie.

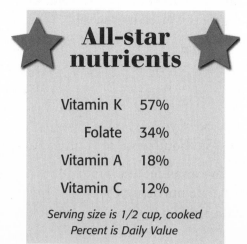

All-star nutrients

Vitamin K	57%
Folate	34%
Vitamin A	18%
Vitamin C	12%

Serving size is 1/2 cup, cooked
Percent is Daily Value

Folate. This B vitamin may help prevent two types of cancer.

■ According to the American Cancer Society, cancer of the pancreas is one of the leading causes of cancer deaths in the United States. Fortunately, a large European study has found that getting lots of folate from your diet lowers your risk of this cancer. However, large amounts of folate from supplements does not.

■ One new study suggests that low blood levels of folate might protect against colon cancer while another shows how low folate levels could trigger cancer-starting changes. More research may help resolve this controversy, so get the latest news from your doctor. But don't stop eating asparagus. It also contains another nutrient that may help foil colon cancer — fructooligosaccharides (FOS).

FOS. Your body doesn't digest fructooligosaccharides like other nutrients. Instead, bacteria in your colon use this nutrient to make the fatty acid butyrate. Together, FOS and butyrate may help trigger several processes that keep colon cancer from developing.

Vitamin C. This antioxidant vitamin can jump in and block the formation of cancer-causing substances like nitrosamines in foods. It can even prevent these compounds from forming in your stomach if you have enough vitamin C in your stomach acid. That's how vitamin C may help reduce your danger of stomach cancer.

Dynamic duo defends your eyes. Asparagus has two nutrients that can help spare your eyes from night blindness, cataracts, macular degeneration, and more.

Vitamin A. It may be more important for your vision than you realize, especially if you've had intestinal surgery or surgery for obesity. According to a Baylor University report, these surgeries can limit your ability to absorb vitamin A, even if the surgery was done long ago. So if you experience vision loss or night blindness, talk to your doctor about possible vitamin A deficiency.

Meanwhile, eat foods like asparagus for added vitamin A. This valuable nutrient helps keep your eyes working properly. Vitamin A's antioxidant power may also help protect your retina from the free radical damage that may eventually lead to cataracts, macular degeneration, night blindness and other vision problems.

■ ■ ■ ■ ■ **Boost the benefits** ■ ■ ■ ■ ■

For added flavor and nutrition, toss steamed asparagus spears with a mix of olive oil and lemon juice. Asparagus gives you vitamin A, vitamin K, lutein, zeaxanthin, and lycopene — all "fat-soluble" nutrients. That means you absorb more of these health-building compounds if you eat them with a little fat — like the healthy fats in olive oil. As a bonus, you'll also get an extra splash of vitamin K from the olive oil itself.

Glutathione. The amino acid glutathione is also a free-radical-fighting antioxidant. In fact, cataracts are more likely when you don't have enough glutathione in your eyes. Fortunately, asparagus is a top source of glutathione — especially if you eat it raw. Plus, the high vitamin C in asparagus may help your body bulk up your glutathione levels.

Toughen your bones against osteoporosis. You could end up with rickety bones if you don't get enough vitamin K. Here's why. A key ingredient in hard-to-break bones is a special protein called osteocalcin. Your body can make this protein without vitamin K, but this underpowered osteocalcin won't help create sturdy bones. Instead, you'll form softer bone that's more easily broken.

But if you get enough vitamin K, your body mixes up a mightier form of osteocalcin, the kind that helps build strong bones. Asparagus can be a big help because just a half cup of cooked asparagus — around 6 spears — gives you more than half the daily vitamin K you need.

Just remember, if you take warfarin or any other blood-thinning medicine, talk to your doctor before adding more vitamin K to your diet. Vitamin K is a blood thinner, too.

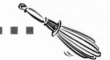

■ ■ ■ ■ *Cook's corner* ■ ■ ■ ■

- The peak season for asparagus flavor and bargains is March through June.

- Fresh asparagus bunches squeak when you squeeze them. Choose spears with far more green coloring than white.

- Before you cook or store asparagus, bend each spear until it breaks. Then throw out the pale, dry lower stem.

- Wrap cut asparagus stems in a damp paper towel or stick them in a glass of water. Slip that arrangement into a plastic bag, and store it in the refrigerator for up to three days.

- Asparagus goes well with dill, olive oil, basil, caraway, chervil, tarragon, or lemon.

Bok choy

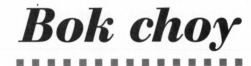

Enjoy the double features of Chinese cabbage

Some say bok choy is two veggies in one, while others say it's a great way to get cabbage benefits without the cabbage taste. That's because the thick stalks of bok choy taste more like lettuce even though the leaves' flavor may still remind you of cabbage.

Not only does bok choy taste different from cabbage, it also looks different. In fact, the white base and stalks are shaped like celery while the tops are leafy and green. But bok choy is still a member of the cabbage family and delivers the same powerful nutritional punch against cancer and other threats to your health.

Recruit five mighty cancer defenders. Bok choy is a star cancer-fighter just like other members of the cabbage family — and here are five reasons why you should try it.

Dithiolethiones. Bok choy guards you with mighty phytochemicals like dithiolethiones to help stop cancer before it starts. These tongue-twisting phytochemicals may not be well known, but they help keep your body's immune system in top form — and that helps block cancer from developing.

Indoles and isothiocyanates. These two I's help thwart cancer in several ways.

- Cancer-causing compounds from foods and other sources can damage your DNA, a scary injury that can turn cells cancerous. But indoles and isothiocyanates help prevent DNA damage.

- Isothiocyanates encourage your body to produce cancer-fighting antioxidants.

- Indoles can help hinder the growth of cancer cells.

And when it comes to destroying cancer-causing compounds, dithiolthiones, indoles, and isothiocyanates all pitch in.

Beta carotene. Bok choy also contains hefty amounts of this cancer-preventing phytochemical. In fact, your body can make lots of vitamin A from that beta carotene. That's why bok choy is known as a leading source of vitamin A. But that's not all.

Experts think beta carotene may give you extra cancer protection. A recent study found that women who got either 12 milligrams (mg) beta carotene

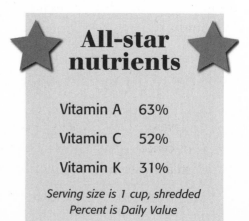

All-star nutrients

Vitamin A   63%

Vitamin C   52%

Vitamin K   31%

Serving size is 1 cup, shredded
Percent is Daily Value

supplement or 4 mg each of beta carotene, lycopene, and lutein experienced less DNA damage. A cup of raw bok choy provides close to 2 mg of beta carotene, but little or no lycopene or lutein. So eat bok choy, but also enjoy lycopene from tomato sauces and tomato soup and lutein from leafy greens like spinach.

Omega-3 fatty acids. Eating foods like bok choy could help lower your risk of cancer in one more way. Experts say omega-6 fatty acids help promote cancer while omega-3 fatty acids battle against it. But the average American's diet is rich in the wrong type of fats. To raise your supply of good fats, consider bok choy, which provides more omega-3s than omega-6s. You'll need other foods to help completely turn the tide, but bok choy is a good place to start.

Vitamin duo battles osteoarthritis. Bok choy, with its high vitamin C and K content, could help you win the war against osteoarthritis.

Vitamin C is a key ingredient in the collagen that makes your cartilage resilient. Research suggests that a high C intake can help slow the progress of osteoarthritis and lessen knee pain. What's more, bok choy's vitamin K may help stop your symptoms from getting worse. One study showed that people with lower levels of vitamin K in their blood were more likely to have bone spurs and other signs of osteoarthritis in their knees and hands. But the higher the levels of vitamin K, the fewer osteoarthritis symptoms the researchers found. So try adding more vitamin C and K to your diet, and give yourself extra protection from osteoarthritis.

Just remember, if you take warfarin or another blood-thinning drug, talk to your doctor before eating bok choy or other foods high in vitamin K.

■ ■ ■ ■ ■ **Boost the benefits** ■ ■ ■ ■ ■

Never boil bok choy. Boiling leaches away large amounts of cancer-fighting phytochemicals. Stir-fry, microwave, or steam your bok choy instead.

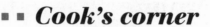

■ ■ ■ ■ *Cook's corner* ■ ■ ■ ■

Choose the right cabbage. Bok choy is one of several Chinese cabbages. It may be labeled as Chinese cabbage, pak-choi, or many other names. Your best bet is to look for a cabbage with stalks and leafy greens. Otherwise you may accidentally buy pe-tsai, another "Chinese cabbage" that's not as nutritious.

Find the freshest. Check for thick, plump, firm stalks and crisp, whole, green leaves.

Keep in the crisper. Store unwashed bok choy in a perforated bag in the fridge for up to two days.

Prep before you cook. Trim the base, separate the stalks as you would celery, and trim the leaves. Wash leaves and stems in cold water right before use.

Eat both treats. Add the raw leaves and stalks to salads, or stir-fry the stalks.

Get your money's worth from organic food

Imagine spending less money but getting even more bang for your organic buck. You can — once you know the truth about organic shopping.

Don't be fooled by labels. When you think of organic, you probably expect an item that was produced with little or no pesticides, herbicides, chemical fertilizers, antibiotics, hormones, additives, or preservatives. But the only items that fit that definition are products labeled "100 percent organic."

An "organic" label means 95 percent of the ingredients are required to be organic. On the other hand, if the label says "made with organic ingredients" only 70 percent is fully organic. In that case, you may not be getting what you pay for. Sometimes, the non-organic ingredients are added vitamins or other nutrients, but they may also be ingredients you'd rather avoid. Look for the USDA organic seal to be sure you're getting the quality you're looking for.

Some produce is already low-pesticide. An unpeeled banana may have pesticide residues, but throw out the peel and the suspicious chemicals go with it. So paying extra for an organic banana may be a waste of money. Other low-pesticide produce include asparagus, broccoli, avocado, pineapple, kiwi, mango, and papaya. Onions, cabbage, frozen peas, and frozen corn may also be nearly pesticide-free.

Spend your money on the top offenders. The "dirty dozen" are fruits and veggies that are highest in pesticide residues. Buy the organic versions of these foods, and you'll be probably get the most for your money. They include potatoes, bell peppers, spinach, celery, raspberries, strawberries, cherries, grapes, peaches, nectarines, apples, and pears.

Broccoli sprouts

■ ■

Surprising power from broccoli tots

If you like the lively taste of radishes but want even more powerful nutrition, broccoli sprouts are the treat you've been waiting for. Regular broccoli seeds are the source of these little sprouts. Yet while regular broccoli is allowed to grow for months, broccoli sprouts are picked and eaten while they're just days old. But don't let their youthful appearance fool you. These sprouts can be weapons of wellness. In fact, they can reduce cholesterol and high blood pressure, and even deliver some cancer protection.

Broccoli was bred from cabbages by the ancient Etruscans of Italy. So like cabbage, broccoli and broccoli sprouts are members of the cancer-fighting *Brassica* family. That's probably why broccoli sprouts contain mighty anti-cancer phytochemicals like sulforaphane. What's more, scientists from Johns Hopkins University have developed special broccoli sprouts — called Broccosprouts — that may supply up to 50 times more sulforaphane than broccoli. That's a lot of power dedicated to defending your health. So just add this common food to your salads, snack bags, or lunch plates — and know you've made a great choice for your health.

Protect yourself with two potent cancer fighters. Sulforaphane and selenium help make broccoli sprouts an amazing weapon against cancer.

Scientists once thought sulforaphane had only one way to fight cancer, but today they suspect sulforaphane may fend off cancer in up to six ways. Consider these examples.

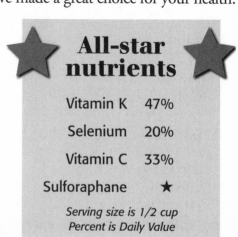

All-star nutrients

Vitamin K	47%
Selenium	20%
Vitamin C	33%
Sulforaphane	★

Serving size is 1/2 cup
Percent is Daily Value

▪ ▪ ▪ ▪ ▪ Boost the benefits ▪ ▪ ▪ ▪ ▪

Eat broccoli sprouts or broccoli with a dash of healthy fat like olive oil, and your body will get more vitamin K. That's because your body needs fat to help you absorb as much of this vitamin as possible.

Avoid boiling broccoli or broccoli sprouts. Boiling leaches out the sulforaphane. Get more sulforaphane by choosing cooking methods like steaming or microwaving instead.

- Sulforaphane is different from antioxidants like vitamin C. Regular antioxidants must sacrifice themselves to deactivate disease-causing molecules in your body, but sulforaphane triggers your body's phase 2 detoxification enzymes. These enzymes rev up your immune system to trap and throw out cancer-causing substances — and the effect lasts longer than protection from antioxidants.

- Sulforaphane also helps wipe out *H. pylori* bacteria in your stomach. These bacteria are known causes of not only stomach cancer, but also ulcers and gastritis. Yet studies show that eating broccoli sprouts helps reduce or eliminate these malicious microbes. So you could lower your risk of stomach cancer and more with ease. On top of that, animal research suggests sulforaphane might prevent tumors in other parts of your body, too.

- Eating broccoli sprouts also helps you get enough selenium in your diet. That's good news because you need selenium to help repair damaged cells before they can turn cancerous. Cancer rates are higher in areas where selenium deficiency is more likely — China, for example — so avoiding selenium deficiency with a little help from broccoli sprouts could be a smart move.

If your supermarket doesn't carry broccoli sprouts, pile your cart with broccoli instead. One leading expert suggests broccoli may prevent cancer just as well as broccoli sprouts. Although sprouts may have more sulforaphane, broccoli has more indoles, a different type of cancer fighter. These mighty phytochemicals may also help you avoid several kinds of cancer.

Get heart smart with sprouts. Hardening of the arteries, high blood pressure, high cholesterol, and damage to your blood vessels can all put your heart at risk, but nutrients in broccoli sprouts can defend you. Here's how.

- Experts suspect vitamin K may help prevent hardening of the arteries. They believe a special protein may shield your arteries from hardening and prevent damaged areas from getting worse, but that protein needs vitamin K to get the job done. A study at the Tufts University Vitamin K Laboratory will soon find out for sure, so stay tuned.

- Research suggests the vitamin C in broccoli sprouts may strengthen your blood vessels and help lower high blood pressure.

- A small Japanese study found that eating 100 grams of broccoli sprouts (around 2 cups) every day for a week helped lower "bad" LDL cholesterol. The sulforaphane in sprouts may also crank up antioxidants to protect your heart and blood vessels even more.

If you don't like broccoli sprouts, fully-grown broccoli is still a good choice. Not only does it have vitamins C and K like broccoli sprouts, it also has extra folate and fiber. Folate helps prevent artery damage by lowering unhealthy homocysteine levels in your blood. Meanwhile, the fiber in broccoli helps your body get rid of more cholesterol.

Warning: sprouts can make you sick

Broccoli sprouts and seeds can become contaminated by bacteria like *Salmonella* and *E. Coli*. Protect yourself by cooking sprouts well, particularly for older adults, children, and people with weakened immune systems. Buy only refrigerated sprouts and store them in your fridge at home. And don't grow your own sprouts — you could get food poisoning from contaminated seeds.

Regardless of whether you choose broccoli or broccoli sprouts, remember this. If you take warfarin or another blood thinner, don't fill up on broccoli or broccoli sprouts without your doctor's permission. Otherwise, the extra vitamin K could cause problems with your medication.

Save your sight from eye diseases. Amazing test tube research suggests the sulforaphane in broccoli sprouts could help protect your vision.

Doctors say ultraviolet light from sunlight damages cells in your eyes. Over the years, enough damage can accumulate to cause macular degeneration or other problems that can lead to blindness. But exciting laboratory research suggests the sulforaphane in broccoli sprouts could make a difference. When researchers exposed samples of retina cells to ultraviolet light, samples treated with sulforaphane proved more likely to survive. What's more, the researchers think sulforaphane might help reduce damage to your eyes for several days at a time.

What mature broccoli lacks in sulforaphane, it makes up with the vision-defending phytochemical lutein. Lutein has rapidly become famous for its potential to slash your danger of cataracts and macular degeneration.

▪ ▪ ▪ ▪ *Cook's corner* ▪ ▪ ▪ ▪

Seek out perfect sprouts. Check your supermarket's produce section for broccoli sprouts. Don't buy any that smell bad, seem mushy, or don't look crisp and fresh.

Store smartly. Keep broccoli sprouts in the refrigerator for up to two weeks. But store unwashed broccoli in a sealed container in the crisper for no more than four days.

Clean up their act. Before eating or cooking broccoli sprouts, rinse them thoroughly and squeeze them in a paper towel.

Serve your sprouts. Add broccoli sprouts to sandwiches, salads, or soups.

Good foods that threaten your health

Vegetables are usually health heroes, but if you have certain conditions, they can actually become health villains. Here's what you need to know if you have one of these health problems or are worried about getting them.

Osteoporosis or kidney stones. Oxalate-rich foods can temporarily prevent you from absorbing calcium, so if you're concerned about osteoporosis, you should try to avoid them. And if you're at high risk for kidney stones — or you've already had one — talk to your doctor about whether oxalates are off limits. Oxalate is a key ingredient in kidney stones, so you may need to limit or avoid foods with a high content. Be particularly wary of these top offenders — spinach, beets, soy products, coffee, cola, nuts, chocolate, tea, wheat bran, strawberries, and rhubarb.

Thyroid problems. Veggie compounds called goitrogens could make things worse for you if you have hypothyroidism because they interfere with the thyroid's hormone-making process. You'll need to limit rutabagas, turnips, cabbage, kale, cauliflower, broccoli, mustard, peanuts, pine nuts, soybeans and soy products, and millet. One thing that may help is cooking them — it appears to lower the amount of goitrogens in the food.

Gout. If gout is your problem, eating high-purine foods may make you feel worse. So avoid the following triggers — scallops, mussels, anchovies, sardines, herring, codfish, trout, haddock, fish roe (eggs), gravy and consommé, turkey, bacon, organ meats like liver and kidneys, veal, and alcohol. You'll find lesser amounts of purines in asparagus, cauliflower, kidney beans, lentils, lima beans, mushrooms, navy beans, peas, and spinach. Early research suggests purines from these foods may turn out to be less worrisome.

Brussels sprouts

■ ■

Big nutrition in a small package

In England, no Christmas dinner is complete unless it includes Brussels sprouts. Although these nutritious little cabbages may have gotten their start in Brussels, Belgium, they've clearly become popular in other nations, too. The Germans call them "rose cabbages," and Thomas Jefferson found some in Paris two centuries ago. In 1812 he began raising his own Brussels sprouts in Virginia — and these small cabbages have been big news ever since.

Like other crucifers, Brussels sprouts are high in vitamin K and vitamin C as well as sulforaphane and other antioxidants. If you cook them properly, you will be rewarded with a side dish that is both tasty and nutritious.

Triple your threat against cancer. The secret of Brussels sprouts is out. These mini-cabbages defend you from cancer just like their larger cousins. And just as you might use several tricks to keep pests out of your garden, Brussels sprouts have at least three "tricks" to keep cancer away from you.

Brussels sprouts deliver two phytochemicals to your cells — indole-3-carbinol (I3C) and sulforaphane. Both help trigger your phase-2 detoxification enzymes, powerful compounds that rev up your body's defense system to evict cancer-causing substances. It's a little like spraying your plants with something bugs dislike.

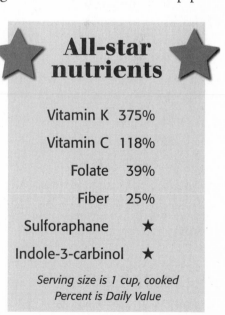

All-star nutrients

Vitamin K	375%
Vitamin C	118%
Folate	39%
Fiber	25%
Sulforaphane	★
Indole-3-carbinol	★

Serving size is 1 cup, cooked
Percent is Daily Value

I3C also changes how estrogen works with your body chemistry — even if you're a man. That's important because estrogen may play a role in several types of cancer. In fact, one small study showed that women who took I3C supplements were more likely to reverse precancerous changes in their cervical cells.

But supplements may not be wise. Preliminary animal studies suggest that taking I3C supplements might raise the risk of cancer especially after exposure to a cancer-causing substance. More research is needed. But meanwhile, eating more Brussels sprouts and similar veggies may be your best bet.

Brussels sprouts are also a rich source of a compound that turns into a tongue-twisting "cancer repellent" called allyl isothiocyanate (AITC). AITC helps prevent regular cells from becoming cancerous.

■ ■ ■ ■ ■ **Boost the benefits** ■ ■ ■ ■ ■

Mushy, boiled Brussels sprouts don't just taste and smell bad. Boiling can cut the cancer-fighting nutrients by up to nearly 60 percent. So instead of boiling, lightly cook your Brussels sprouts by stir frying them or steaming them. They'll be deliciously nourishing and stench-free.

If you avoid Brussels sprouts because they give you gas, put them into boiling water for 1 minute and then drop them into ice water for 1 minute. Remove them from the water quickly and then cook them.

Step up your Alzheimer's defenses. You may not think of Brussels sprouts when you think of Alzheimer's prevention, but their folate might actually cut your odds.

Past research suggested folate might not affect memory or Alzheimer's risk, but a new study found three years of folate supplements helped people with high blood levels of homocysteine by improving memory and speed of information processing. High homocysteine has been associated with both heart disease and Alzheimer's, but folate helps reduce it.

Although the study used 800-milligram supplements, you can get almost as much folate from this combo — a half cup of Special K or Product 19 cereal for breakfast plus a half-cup of rice and a cup of Brussels sprouts later in the day. Just make sure you get enough vitamin B12 when adding folate because studies show a high-folate, low-B12 combination impairs brain processes, including memory and learning. What's more, older adults may not absorb enough vitamin B12 from foods, so talk to your doctor about whether you're getting enough. In the meantime, add more B12 with foods like clam chowder, Special K, or Product 19.

Pick vitamins to stop osteoporosis. Making strong bone without all the right ingredients is like trying to make a bulletproof vest out of lace. It may look good, but it won't protect you. That's why you not only need calcium and vitamin D to keep strong bones, but vitamin C and vitamin K as well.

Your skeleton constantly rebuilds itself by casting off old bone and forming fresh bone to replace it. To make this new bone tough, you need compounds called osteocalcin and collagen. But your body must have vitamin C to produce collagen and vitamin K to make osteocalcin that's not brittle. Fortunately, Brussels sprouts can help you make a good start on getting enough of these bone-building vitamins.

■ ■ ■ ■ *Cook's corner* ■ ■ ■ ■

Choose smaller sprouts that are bright green, firm, and have tightly packed leaves. Brussels sprouts are in season from October through March.

Store unwashed sprouts in the fridge for up to four days. Just before cooking, rinse them with water, strip any yellowed or wilted leaves, and trim off most of the stem end. Don't cut right down to the base or leaves will drop off during cooking.

To check whether sprouts have finished cooking, insert a knife in the base of a sprout. A sprout that is just slightly tender is done.

Spice sprouts with thyme, paprika, or sage.

Butternut squash

Great reasons to fall for a winter wonder

"Why do you build me up, butternut baby, when I feel run-down ..." Maybe that's not exactly how the song goes, but butternut squash can help build up your health because it's chock full of powerful nutrition. Not only is this squash loaded with vitamins C and A, it also has B vitamins, manganese, vitamin E, and other remarkable nutrients.

Yet, butternut squash isn't just good for you. This ancient food from Mexico is also sweet and delicious. In fact, Australians even call it the "butternut pumpkin" because of its pumpkin-like taste. What's more, butternut squash is such a close relative of the pumpkin you can substitute it for pumpkin in recipes.

So look for this yummy, long-necked squash during the cool weather months. You'll recognize it by its gold-kissed beige color and its unique round-bottomed vase shape.

Win the war against arthritis. Around 7 million people in

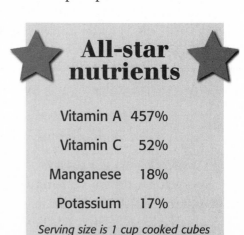

All-star nutrients

Vitamin A	457%
Vitamin C	52%
Manganese	18%
Potassium	17%

Serving size is 1 cup cooked cubes
Percent is Daily Value

the United States battle the pain of rheumatoid arthritis (RA), but you don't have to become one of them. Eating delicious butternut squash regularly can give you two powerful arthritis preventers — vitamin C and beta cryptoxanthin.

> ▪▪▪▪▪ **Boost the benefits** ▪▪▪▪▪
>
> Baking a butternut squash makes it taste oh-so-much sweeter, plus it preserves all the valuable beta carotene. But think carefully before you try boiling your squash. Boiling leeches out both flavor and nutrients.

According to Mayo Clinic research, beta cryptoxanthin is an antioxidant that may help lower your risk of rheumatoid arthritis. Others things that might lower RA risk include fruits and cruciferous veggies, like cabbage, and the mineral zinc.

On top of that, beta cryptoxanthin and vitamin C may help prevent RA by defending your body against another form of arthritis called inflammatory polyarthritis — the inflammation of more than one joint. Research suggests people who develop inflammatory polyarthritis may be more likely to get rheumatoid arthritis later.

But getting the right nutrients may help. An English study found that people who got the least vitamin C from their diets have three times as much risk of inflammatory polyarthritis. And another study suggests that people who eat the most foods rich in beta cryptoxanthin are at less risk of inflammatory polyarthritis.

Start avoiding arthritis with butternut squash and other rich sources of vitamin C and beta cryptoxanthin — like sweet red peppers and orange juice.

Squelch a stroke with squash power. Even if you're already taking diuretics for high blood pressure, you can still lower your risk of stroke. A study from the Queen's Medical Center in Hawaii found that people who ate the least potassium had a higher risk of stroke even if they already took diuretics. A recent review of research confirms that eating plenty of foods high in potassium lowers your stroke risk. What's more, eating potassium rich-produce slashes your risk of dying from a stroke if you ever have one. And that's not all.

Butternut squash is also a good source of magnesium. Since magnesium deficiency has been linked to stroke, you can't afford to scrimp. Learn to love butternut squash but add extra sources of potassium, like baked potatoes, white beans, dates, and lima beans, as well as magnesium-rich foods, like halibut, spinach, and black beans.

Scare off a cluster of cancers. You might not know it yet, but butternut squash is a triple-threat against 10 different kinds of cancer. That's because it supplies you with three powerful cancer fighters — vitamin A, beta carotene, and vitamin C.

Research shows a shortage of vitamin A may raise your risk of cancer, but a cup of butternut squash cubes delivers your daily recommended amount of vitamin A and then some. The squash's secret is its treasure trove of beta carotene, which your body turns into cancer-blocking vitamin A.

Even better, getting enough beta carotene and vitamin C may cut your risk of a number of cancers — colon, esophagus, stomach, pancreatic, lung, rectal, prostate, breast, ovarian, and cervix. Don't forget that a cup of butternut squash cubes is a great start on your vitamin C for the day, and it has all the daily beta carotene experts recommend.

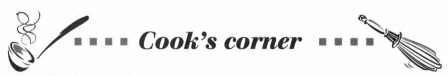

▪ ▪ ▪ ▪ *Cook's corner* ▪ ▪ ▪ ▪

Store raw, whole butternut squash for up to a month in a well-ventilated, partly humid, dark place where temperatures linger in the 50s (Fahrenheit.) Do not remove the stem before use. Store cut or cooked squash in your refrigerator for a couple of days.

To avoid the work of peeling your squash, cut it in half, scoop out any seeds and strings, and bake one half squash for 30 to 40 minutes at 400 degrees. Discard the skin after eating the delicate flavored interior.

Be a smart shopper. A 2001 report named winter squash as one of the foods most likely to be contaminated by pesticides and other harmful chemicals. If you're concerned about this, buy organic butternut squash. Purchase from a local organic grower in season, and you may find a good price.

Cabbage

A head start on better health

Cabbage has been saving lives and making history for centuries. The cabbage dish called sauerkraut helped Asian workers build the Great Wall of China. Cabbage also kept sailors from dying of scurvy during Captain Cook's voyage to the Antarctic Circle. It even helped northern Europeans survive harsh winters during the Middle Ages. But long before any of that, the ancient Roman, Cato the Elder, recommended crushed cabbage leaves to treat cancerous ulcers. He was on the

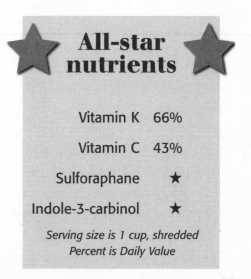

All-star nutrients

Vitamin K   66%

Vitamin C   43%

Sulforaphane   ★

Indole-3-carbinol   ★

Serving size is 1 cup, shredded
Percent is Daily Value

right track. Modern science confirms that cabbage is an easy but power-ful way to help prevent cancer.

Choose from regular green cabbage, crinkle-leaved Savoy, or delight-ful red cabbage. All are nutritious and delicious in stir-fries, salads, and more. Just be careful with cole slaw. The ones made with mayonnaise could deliver more fat and calories than you want.

■ ■ ■ ■ ■ **Boost the benefits** ■ ■ ■ ■ ■

Get rid of all the things you hate about cabbage, and make it more nutritious, too. First, try sweet-tasting Napa cabbage in place of regular cabbage for gentler flavor and extra vitamin C. Next, prevent smelly, limp cabbage by chopping or shredding it into small pieces and cook-ing it no longer than five minutes. If you quickly steam or stir-fry cabbage instead of boiling it, you could retain up to 60 percent more of its cancer-fighting nutrients.

Get cabbage fever and cut cancer risk. Find new ways to enjoy cab-bage, and you could add extra muscle to your cancer defense. Here's how.

Some cancer-causing substances don't make trouble until a special enzyme "switches on" their ability to damage cells and DNA. But cabbage contains an isothiocyanate called benzyl isothiocyanate (BITC). Animal studies suggest that BITC may stop most enzymes from flipping the "on switch" so your cells are more likely to escape cancer-causing damage.

But cabbage doesn't just take out inactive cancer-causers. It also delivers sulforaphane to combat cancer-causing substances that are already active. Sulforaphane persuades your liver to produce more of its potent phase-2 detoxification enzymes. These extra shock troops super-charge your immune system, arming it with more power to disarm cancer-causing substances and sweep them out of your body.

Like sulforaphane, the indole-3-carbinol (I3C) in cabbage also helps marshal your phase-2 enzymes against cancer danger. But that's not all.

I3C also helps keep the estrogen in your body from becoming a trigger for cancer. Even so, you may not want to try I3C supplements just yet. Animal studies suggest I3C supplements might raise the risk of cancer. Future research will determine whether supplements are dangerous to people, but meanwhile get your I3C from cabbages rather than capsules.

Eat red cabbage and you may even get a little extra benefit if you're a woman past menopause. Red cabbage has up to 28 times more flavonoids than other cabbages, and one study found that women who ate more flavonoids lowered their breast cancer risk. To make sure you get enough of these healthful flavonoids, enjoy cabbage along with other treats like apples, broccoli, tea, and onions.

Sauerkraut — a potent cancer fighter

You may turn your nose up at sauerkraut, but this form of cabbage can defend your health just as well as its full-leaf counterpart. Research suggests that eating sauerkraut, raw cabbage, or quick-cooked cabbage three times a week may lower women's risk of breast cancer, particularly if they started eating it when they were younger. What's more, a Finnish study found that turning white cabbage into sauerkraut creates cancer-fighting isothiocyanates. If you're on a low-salt diet, strain and rinse canned sauerkraut before eating it — or just eat more raw or short-cooked cabbage.

Dodge gum disease and save your heart. Most people think they're safe from tooth-stealing gum disease, but estimates suggest 50 percent of Americans have mild gum disease and nearly a third have periodontitis, the more serious kind of gum disease. Oddly enough, cabbage may be able to help, thanks to its surprising payload of vitamin C.

Along with good dental hygiene and calcium-rich foods, some dental specialists now recommend vitamin C for healthy gums and teeth. That's because research shows that people who don't get enough vitamin C have a higher risk of gum disease. Fortunately eating just a few ounces of shredded cabbage can give you as much C as a half cup of pineapple.

But there's more. A 2005 study found a link between periodontitis and the clogged arteries that can lead to a heart attack. More studies are needed, but for now, eat more cabbage — especially Savoy cabbage which has extra vitamin C. To be sure you don't come up short, eat cabbage along with other vitamin C-rich foods like sweet peppers and citrus fruits.

Crucifer helps you say bye to bruises. You've just found yet another "black and blue," and you can't imagine how you got it. If you're bruising more easily than you once did, check your diet and medications. One of them could be lowering your levels of vitamin K — which could be why you're "cruising for a bruising."

Think about it. Easy bruising is a symptom of vitamin K deficiency, and medications like antibiotics, mineral oil, cholestyramine, or orlistat can help cause it. Even frequent use of aspirin can cut your cache of K. What's more, conditions like diarrhea or liver disease can also sap your body's supply of this critical vitamin. So if you bruise more easily than you did last year, ask your doctor what to do about it. Meanwhile, enjoy more cabbage, leafy greens, and other delicious foods rich in vitamin K.

But be careful. If you take warfarin or another blood-thinning medication, never add more vitamin K to your diet without asking your doctor first.

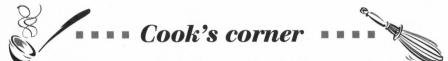

▪ ▪ ▪ ▪ *Cook's corner* ▪ ▪ ▪ ▪

Choose a fine specimen. Look for crisp-leaved cabbage heads that feel heavy for their size. Avoid any cabbage with discolored or soft spots.

Plan a-head. Keep raw, uncut cabbage in a sealed plastic bag in your refrigerator for up to 10 days.

Prep for use. Before cooking or eating, wash the cabbage and cut out its core.

Turn up the taste. Spice cabbage with oregano, dill, celery seed, caraway, or savory.

Keep seeing red. Add vinegar or lemon juice to red cabbage when cooking or cutting it. Otherwise, it may turn blue or purple.

Carrots

■ ■ ■ ■ ■ ■ ■ ■ ■ ■ ■

Your 'root' to 24-karat health

The original carrot wasn't orange when it first appeared in Afghanistan centuries ago. Instead, it was purple on the outside and yellow inside. Nearly a thousand years passed before the Dutch introduced an orange carrot to the world. But unusually colored carrots are making a comeback. The U.S. Department of Agriculture has developed yellow, purple, and red carrots that have extra phytochemicals like lutein and lycopene. Even their newest orange carrot has 30 percent more beta carotene.

But the standard carrot still has plenty to offer. Next to beets, carrots are the sweetest veggie you can eat. They also give you vibrant phytochemicals like alpha carotene, beta carotene, and beta cryptoxanthin so your body can make vitamin A. Scientists have even discovered a surprising new nutrient in carrots that can help keep you healthier longer.

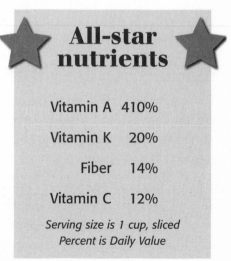

All-star nutrients

Vitamin A 410%

Vitamin K 20%

Fiber 14%

Vitamin C 12%

Serving size is 1 cup, sliced
Percent is Daily Value

■ ■ ■ ■ ■ **Boost the benefits** ■ ■ ■ ■ ■

To keep more nutrition in your carrots, scrub them clean instead of peeling them. You may want to peel them anyway if they're old or discolored.

Cooking your carrots with a little added fat will help you get the most beta carotene. Fat helps your body absorb this nutrient, and cooking allows the fat and beta carotene to mix better, so you absorb even more. But try not to use boiling as your cooking method. Boiling robs your carrots of most of the nutrient falcarinol.

Smart way to declare war on cancer. Any time you hear Bugs Bunny say, "What's up doc," he's probably eating a carrot. And that's not a bad idea because carrots add three weapons to your tumor-prevention arsenal.

Exciting research from England suggests carrots may deliver a new cancer fighter, a compound called falcarinol. Scientists found that animals whose diets were supplemented with either falcarinol alone or raw carrots were one-third less likely to develop colon tumors than animals on a standard diet. Although no one knows whether falcarinol protects people the same way, the study's lead researcher recommends eating one small carrot every day.

Yet carrots don't just give you falcarinol. They're also a super source of vitamin A because your body turns their alpha carotene and beta carotene into vitamin A. In fact, a Swedish study discovered that people who ate the most carotenes and vitamin A were less likely to get stomach cancer. And a study of people in their 70s found that those with the highest blood levels of beta carotene had a lower risk of dying — especially from cancer.

Just remember, the source of your beta carotene may be important. A few studies have suggested beta carotene supplements might raise your risk of lung cancer, while other research disagrees. However, another study found that high blood levels of beta carotene might be linked to more risk of aggressive prostate cancer. That study's researchers say you should be cautious about taking beta carotene supplements.

Still, studies have found that diets rich in beta carotene and vitamin A cut your odds of many kinds of cancer. So skip the supplements, and make an effort to get your beta carotene from delicious orange foods like carrots, sweet potatoes, apricots, and pumpkins.

Beat high cholesterol with a (carrot) stick. You might not expect carrots to help fight cholesterol, but these crunchy veggies will surprise you. In fact, carrots have two potential ways to help you cut high cholesterol.

All carrots contain soluble fiber, including a kind called calcium pectate. Research shows this remarkable fiber can help shave your cholesterol — shaving your heart attack risk right along with it. On top of that, the beta carotene in carrots may help your cholesterol levels, too. Scientists found that rats whose diets were supplemented with dried carrot for three weeks absorbed less cholesterol than rats on a standard diet. Until researchers determine whether beta carotene works the same way in humans, eating more carrot sticks certainly can't hurt — and it may give you bonus protection beyond just cutting your cholesterol.

Your "bad" LDL cholesterol turns even more dangerous when harmful molecules called free radicals attack your body. Free radicals help turn LDL cholesterol into artery-clogging plaque. Over time, repeated free-radical attacks help build up so much plaque that it blocks the blood flow to your heart and causes a heart attack. But carrots have vitamin C to help prevent that. This intrepid vitamin helps defend your LDL cholesterol from free radical attacks, so plaque is less likely to build up and put you in danger. Just be sure to get additional vitamin C from foods like sweet peppers and citrus fruits.

And if you're ever tempted to skip eating carrots, remember this. Early research suggests the high vitamin K in carrots may also help prevent hardening of your arteries.

Eat your way out of night blindness. If you've begun having more trouble seeing and driving at night than you once did, you could have night blindness. This means either you see poorly in dim light or you take longer to recover from the glare of headlights or other lights. Talk to your eye doctor or regular doctor about this as soon as possible, but check your diet, too. Night blindness is an early symptom of vitamin A deficiency. Try eating more carrots and other foods rich in vitamin A, and see if your night vision improves. Sweet potatoes, pumpkin, fortified cereals, and leafy greens are all good choices.

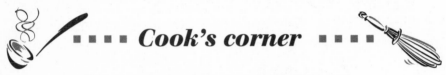

Cook's corner

- Choose carrots that are smooth, firm, and brightly colored. For extra sweetness, pick carrots that are slender rather than thick. Avoid cracks or signs of withering or softening.

- The carrot is actually a tap root meant to draw moisture and vitamins to the green carrot tops. Remove the tops as quickly as possible to keep the vitamins and moisture in the carrot.

- Revive limp carrots. Soak them for 30 minutes in ice water in the fridge to turn them crisp again.

- Store carrots in a sealed plastic bag in the fridge for up to 10 days. But don't keep them close to apples or pears or they'll start to taste bitter.

7 secrets to safer produce

Washing fresh leafy greens and herbs with diluted vinegar before you cook or eat them could save you from food poisoning. Here are seven more tips to help protect you from contaminated produce.

- Start while you shop. Only buy fresh or bagged produce if it is refrigerated or tucked into a bed of ice.

- If you buy pre-cut or already-peeled produce, refrigerate it the moment you get home.

- Check whether your refrigerator is keeping your food cold enough. Visit your local hardware store and ask about a thermometer for fridge temperatures. Make sure your refrigerator is set to 40 degrees Fahrenheit or less.

- Moisture is like a party invitation for food-poisoning bacteria, so don't let greens soak in the sink. Also, don't wash produce if you plan to store it in the fridge a few minutes later.

- Before peeling or eating fruits and veggies, wash them well and then dry them with a clean paper towel.

- Produce with a rind should be scrubbed with a clean brush before peeling. Otherwise, your peeling knife may transfer outside bacteria to the edible inside of your fruit or veggie.

- To destroy *E. coli*, sauté or boil leafy greens at 160 degrees Fahrenheit or higher for at least 15 seconds.

Cauliflower

■■■■■■■■■■■■■■■■■■

Defend your health with 'flower power'

It's true. You're eating a flower when you bite into cauliflower. A cauliflower head is a group of flowers that stopped growing while they were still buds. By that time, the stems leading up to the buds had already begun stockpiling nutrients for the flowers. That's why cauliflower is so nutritious.

You may also be surprised to learn that cauliflower is descended from wild cabbages. But if you could see the cauliflower plant growing, you'd find cabbage-like leaves covering the cauliflower head. Those leaves keep out the sun so cauliflower stays white instead of producing chlorophyll that would turn it green.

Don't be fooled by cauliflower's gentle coloring, mild appearance, or delicate taste. This veggie is a take-no-prisoners fighter that helps keep you healthy.

Splurge on anti-cancer cuisine. Colorful fruits and veggies are your best cancer fighters, but cauliflower is an exception to the rule. Like its cousins, cabbage and broccoli, cauliflower is loaded with some of the most powerful anti-cancer weapons around. Consider these examples.

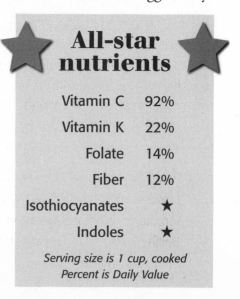

All-star nutrients

Vitamin C	92%
Vitamin K	22%
Folate	14%
Fiber	12%
Isothiocyanates	★
Indoles	★

Serving size is 1 cup, cooked
Percent is Daily Value

■ *Isothiocyanates.* New research from Texas discovered that people who ate the most isothiocyanate-rich foods had almost 30 percent less risk of bladder cancer. That's a great reason to eat more cauliflower, as well as kale, broccoli, cabbage, watercress, and brussels sprouts. An isothiocyanate called phenethyl isothiocyanate helps prevent cells from turning cancerous and even kills existing cancer cells. Sulforaphane, another isothiocyanate, stimulates your liver to produce more special phase 2 detoxification enzymes. These enzymes deliver a long burst of high-voltage power to your immune system so it can neutralize cancer-causing substances and whisk them out of your body.

- *Indole-3-carbinol (I3C).* These amazing phytochemicals raise your count of phase 2 detoxification enzymes, just like sulforaphane. But I3C also helps prevent your body's estrogen from becoming a cancer-causing substance.

- *Folate.* Although two studies suggested folic acid supplements may raise your risk of cancer, getting more of this important B vitamin from food — called folate in its natural form — may slash your risk. According to Harvard researchers, people who get the most folate, vitamin B6, and vitamin B12 from their diets are less likely to develop cancer of the pancreas, but you must keep your weight down to get this benefit. When you eat cauliflower, you'll get a good helping of this important nutrient — without fat or loads of calories. Add rice, clam chowder, chickpeas and cereal to your diet, and you'll not only get more folate, but more B12 and B6, too.

■ ■ ■ ■ ■ Boost the benefits ■ ■ ■ ■ ■

Indian cooks combine cauliflower with pungent spices, like turmeric, and maybe you should, too. Animal research from Rutgers University found that anti-cancer chemicals from cauliflower and turmeric were more effective at slowing the spread of prostate cancer when used together.

Enjoy cauliflower with curry next time. You'll give your cauliflower a little zing, and you'll fortify your body against cancer, too. Just don't make the mistake of boiling your cauliflower. Boiling leaches the cancer-fighting phytochemicals out into the cooking water.

Get hip to new and improved cauliflower

Orange is the color of autumn leaves, pumpkins, and a new kind of cauliflower. Now, you can buy an orange cauliflower that gives you 25 times more beta carotene than standard white cauliflower. Or you can try purple Jacaranda cauliflower. This violet veggie is rich in anthocyanins, the healthy phytochemicals normally found in berries and red wine. You can even "go green" with broccoflower. This child of cancer-fighting broccoli and cauliflower is shaped like regular cauliflower, but you'll see its chartreuse color from a mile away.

Great way to counteract your cataract risk. Only 10 percent of Americans over age 65 think they're at risk for serious vision problems, but more than 50 percent of them have cataracts. Yet, if you're a cauliflower fan, you've already taken a step to lower your cataract risk.

A Japanese study of over 30,000 people found that those who got the most vitamin C in their diets had significantly lower chances of developing cataracts. Cauliflower helps you escape cataracts because it's an excellent source of vitamin C. Other scrumptious sources of this vision-shielding vitamin include sweet peppers, broccoli, and citrus fruits.

Get drug-free help for hemorrhoids. Life without hemorrhoids could be closer than you think. Studies suggest people who take fiber laxatives are only half as likely to have lasting symptoms of hemorrhoids. But you deserve something better than fiber laxatives. After all, they only deliver fiber — not flavor and nutrition.

Cauliflower, on the other hand, is easier to swallow, tastes better, and gives you plenty of fiber and nutrients. So if you're battling hemorrhoids, drink extra water and gradually add more cauliflower and other fiber-filled favorites to your diet.

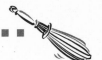

▪▪▪▪ *Cook's corner* ▪▪▪▪

- Choose cauliflower that's firm, tightly packed, and heavy. Avoid cauliflower with black spots or any signs of yellowing or wilting.

- Before cooking cauliflower, remove the leaves, cut out the core, wash the head thoroughly, and pull the florets apart.

- Preserve the color. Avoid cooking cauliflower in aluminum or iron pots. Otherwise, it may turn strange colors.

- Cooking cauliflower for too long is what makes it smell horrid. Either short-cook regular cauliflower or choose broccoflower (green cauliflower), which naturally cooks more quickly and smells better.

- Jazz up cauliflower with chives, curry, turmeric, garlic, ginger, lemon, or mustard seed. Or mix it into your favorite pasta salads and soups.

- Keep unwashed cauliflower in a plastic bag in the fridge for up to one week.

Chili peppers

Vibrant veggie stokes fires of wellness

A chili pepper a day kept trouble away from American Indians. They discovered that burning chili peppers created such caustic fumes invading Europeans kept their distance.

The secret to this defense and the blazing chili pepper taste is capsaicin, a substance found in the skin, seeds, and inner ribs. That's what creates the fire — from mild to wild — in the various kinds of chili peppers.

If you prefer mildly spicy, try the gentle heat of the Anaheim pepper or its spicier cousin, the poblano. After that, the peppers get progressively hotter from the fiery jalapeno to the searing serrano to the blazing cayenne and — for true heat seekers — the twin infernos of the habanero and scotch bonnet peppers.

Just remember, if you're going to cook with chili peppers, it's wiser to use too little than too much.

Hot ticket to hunger-free weight loss. Losing weight used to be a story of hunger pangs, boring food, and misery, but that's all about to change. A Japanese study uncovered a delicious way to eat fewer calories without really trying.

According to the study, people who ate a steaming, spicy soup 10 minutes before their lunch ate fewer calories during lunch. On top of that, those who ate soup that was as spicy as they could comfortably stand also ate fewer fat grams. Another study got similar results with spicy tomato juice 30 minutes before a

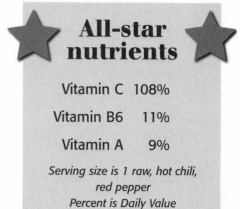

All-star nutrients

Vitamin C 108%

Vitamin B6 11%

Vitamin A 9%

Serving size is 1 raw, hot chili, red pepper
Percent is Daily Value

meal. In both studies, participants ate until they were full, but needed fewer calories to feel satisfied.

Even better, this natural appetite suppressant may last a long time. Canadian researchers report that a pepper-laced breakfast not only reduced hunger all morning, but it also cut the protein and fat people ate at lunch.

Chili peppers might also help you avoid weight gain, thanks to their vitamin C. One researcher suspects low blood levels of vitamin C may cause people to gain more weight over time. And, in fact, a study suggests low vitamin C levels limit your body's ability to burn fat. Another study even associated low blood levels of vitamin C with thicker waists and more body fat.

Scientists still need more evidence to be sure vitamin C influences how much weight you gain or lose. But meanwhile, remember that chili peppers are a leading source of vitamin C. To be sure you get enough of this important vitamin, enjoy other vitamin C-rich foods, like strawberries, watercress, and oranges.

■ ■ ■ ■ ■ Boost the benefits ■ ■ ■ ■ ■

Fresh chili peppers contain more vitamin C than peppers that have been dried, cooked, or canned. They can also be a wonderful addition to sandwiches, pico de gallo, dips, relishes, salad dressing, and salsa.

Of course, chili peppers still serve up plenty of flavor and vitamin A even when they're not fresh and raw. Use them to spice up stews, cornbread, curries, casseroles, or the original "great bowls of fire" — chili. Recipes from Indian, Spanish, Mexican, Cajun, Jamaican, and Oriental cuisines may give you even more tantalizing ways to enjoy chili peppers.

Pit pepper protection against kidney stones. Hot stuff has the right stuff when it comes to avoiding kidney stones. And in this case, the right stuff is vitamin B6. Scientists suspect a deficiency in this vitamin may cause your body to make more oxalate — a key component of painful kidney stones. Some people become deficient because they don't get enough B6 in their diets while other people take medications that cause B6 deficiency. Ask your doctor or pharmacist if you take one of those medications.

Meanwhile, if you're worried about kidney stones, start getting more vitamin B6 from foods. A little chili pepper is a tasty place to start, but you can also find B6 in chickpeas, fortified cereals, and rice.

Forty milligrams of vitamin B6 supplements have been reported to help lower kidney stone risk in women, but talk to your doctor before you try them. Supplements can interfere with some prescription drugs.

Fire up speedier wound healing. If your cuts, scrapes, and other wounds seem to heal too slowly, chili peppers could shorten your road to recovery. Chili peppers are a good source of beta carotene your body can convert to vitamin A. Animal research suggests that both vitamin A and beta carotene can help wounds heal faster — especially if you haven't been getting enough vitamin A from your diet. So spice up your favorite foods with a few extra chili peppers, but don't stop there. Load up on beta carotene and vitamin A from sweet potatoes, carrots, turnip greens, sweet red peppers, kale, pumpkin, and spinach.

Turn up the heat to beat indigestion. Spicy hot food might cool the pain, nausea, and full feeling from indigestion. In a small Italian study, researchers gave study participants two capsules of chili pepper or a placebo before each meal. After two weeks, those who took the chili pepper capsules reported less stomach pain, fullness, and nausea. The capsaicin in chili peppers may be the reason why. The researchers suspect it makes your stomach less sensitive by blocking nerve impulses to the brain.

Try spicing up your food with chili peppers or eating a chili-spiced appetizer before a meal. Just remember two things. Chili peppers can irritate your stomach and may cause indigestion in some people. Don't try peppers if you have gastroesophageal reflux disease (GERD), ulcers, irritable bowel syndrome, or heartburn. Also, don't try substituting black pepper for chili pepper. Black pepper can irritate your stomach.

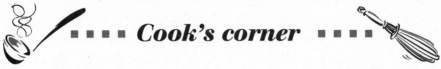

Cook's corner

When that burning in your mouth gets too hot to handle, remember "fire and rice." Rice eases the flames better than most liquids. Other good choices include bread, potatoes, yogurt, or milk.

But the real "fire hazard" may come earlier when you're cleaning, preparing, or cooking your peppers. The seeds and inner ribs of the pepper contain oil that can irritate your skin, eyes, and mouth. So once you cut open a chili, don't touch your mouth, nose, eyes — or any item they'll touch later.

Even washing your hands with soap and water may not remove all the oil, although washing with vinegar may help. Your best bet is to wear rubber or latex gloves or even plastic bags over your hands while working with chili peppers.

Fennel

Rising star makes wellness tastier

If you haven't experienced fennel, you're in for a treat. More Americans are discovering what French and Italian cooks have always known — that fennel is a delicious addition to any meal.

You have two kinds of fennel to choose from — an herb and a vegetable. The herb, common fennel, produces seeds for your spice rack.

Their taste is similar to anise or licorice, but lighter and sweeter. Florence fennel, or finocchio, is a vegetable with an apple-like crunch and milder hints of the sweet flavor in fennel seeds. You'll find this tantalizing taste in both the flavorful bulb and crisp celery-like stalks. Whichever you choose, you'll find powerful nutrients to help you feel better today and protect your health in the future.

Roll those (gall)stones away. By age 60, nearly 25 percent of women have gallstones even if they don't have any symptoms. By age 75, that number soars to 50 percent. Fortunately, vitamin C can help, and fennel is a delightful way to get more of it.

Here's what vitamin C can do. Experts say a build-up of cholesterol in your gallbladder is the reason most people get gallstones. Women may be particularly prone to stones because their estrogen adds more cholesterol to the gallbladder fluids. But the vitamin C in your body helps break down that cholesterol so it won't form stones. In fact, a research study discovered that women with higher blood levels of vitamin C were indeed less likely to have gallstones.

Experiment with fennel, and you'll find a new and delicious way to add more vitamin C to your diet. It could help you dodge the next gallstone — and many more besides.

Beat high blood pressure naturally. One of fennel's older names comes from the word maraino, meaning to grow thin. That's appropriate because fennel's potassium and fiber may help thin down your blood pressure readings over time.

If you're like most Americans, you get twice as much sodium from food as potassium, and that can help raise your blood pressure. Your goal should be to switch them so you're taking in more potassium. In fact, your body needs five times as much potassium as sodium to stay healthy. Eating more potassium-rich foods like fennel not only

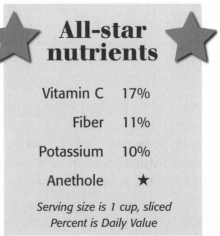

All-star nutrients

Vitamin C	17%
Fiber	11%
Potassium	10%
Anethole	★

*Serving size is 1 cup, sliced
Percent is Daily Value*

helps reduce your blood pressure, but it may also slash your risk of a disabling stroke.

Fiber can also help lower your blood pressure, but it may take eight weeks or longer to work, so be patient. If you take the time to add fiber to your diet gradually and drink plenty of water, you'll avoid gas and other unpleasant side effects. What's more, once you're getting plenty of fiber from produce like fennel, you may lose weight as well — and that could deflate your blood pressure even more.

■ ■ ■ ■ ■ **Boost the benefits** ■ ■ ■ ■ ■

Fennel is a good start on the potassium, vitamin C, and fiber you need each day, but don't stop there. Add more potassium from bananas. Enjoy sweet peppers, strawberries, papayas, and cranberry juice cocktail for added vitamin C. And add both potassium and hearty fiber from foods like beans, raisins, and dates.

Get gas relief from your spice rack. Imagine eating a delicious dinner in India after a day of sightseeing. At the end of your meal, you receive an inviting dish of aromatic fennel seeds to nibble. These seeds are an age-old remedy for indigestion and gas. The secret may be the phytochemical anethole, a compound that relaxes your stomach muscles, speeds up digestion, and prompts your liver to make more bile. Herbal experts say these effects can help relieve gas, indigestion, stomachache, heartburn, and may even ease diarrhea, constipation, and irritable bowel syndrome symptoms.

Before trying fennel, check with your doctor. People taking certain antibiotics shouldn't use fennel. Neither should people with breast cancer, prostate cancer, carrot or celery allergies, or anyone prone to seizures. But if your doctor approves, chew several seeds a few times each day. Or steep a teaspoon of crushed seeds in boiled water for 15 minutes, remove the seeds and drink up. But stay out of the sun while using fennel. It makes your skin more sun-sensitive than usual.

While soothing your stomach, you may also reap some surprise benefits from this remedy.

- Indian research found that fennel seeds have mighty antioxidant power to help your body resist disease.

- Animal studies suggest anethole may help your body fight inflammation and cancer. More research is needed to know for sure, so stay tuned.

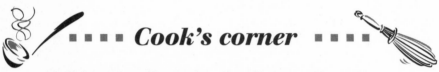

Cook's corner

Pick fennel bulbs that are firm, large, and compact. They should be slightly shiny with a white or green tint, not dry with splits or brown areas. The best stalks also have feathery green fronds.

Get a better value. Pick larger bulbs, and you'll waste less during preparation.

Cut fennel stalks from the base, wrap each separately in plastic wrap, and keep in the fridge for up to four days.

Prepare bulbs perfectly. Trim off a thin slice from the bulb bottom. Pull away the bulb's outer layer and discard. Slice the rest horizontally or vertically, or chop before using. Add fennel bulb or stalk slices to salads, sandwiches, soup, chicken, salmon, or fish dishes. Sauté or steam it as a side dish.

Garlic

■ ■ ■ ■ ■ ■ ■ ■ ■

Tasty bulb lights the way to better health

According to legend, the world's first labor strike was caused by a garlic shortage in ancient Egypt. When the pyramid builders learned their daily garlic ration would be reduced, they simply refused to work. Garlic was that important.

Today's scientists are beginning to see why. They've uncovered a crack team of health-shielding garlic compounds including ajoene, diallyl sulfide (DAS), diallyl disulfide (DADS), and diallyl trisulfide (DATS.) Research suggests these may defend you against cancer, heart attacks, and more. This herb has even been called "Russian penicillin" thanks to its anti-infection powers against bacteria that cause respiratory and digestive infections. In fact, garlic not only kills bacteria, but viruses and infectious fungi, too.

So take your cue from those striking pyramid builders and insist on a daily helping of garlic. You'll find fresh bulbs in your supermarket — each containing up to 24 delectable cloves dedicated to keeping you healthy. Just remember, check with your doctor before adding more garlic to your diet if you take saquinavir or blood thinners like warfarin. Garlic may interact with these medicines.

Defend your heart by playing it smart. Just because a recent study reported garlic doesn't help lower cholesterol, that doesn't mean garlic has no nutrients to help protect your heart. What's more, several experts insist it's too early to give up on garlic. Here are three reasons why you shouldn't give up on garlic either.

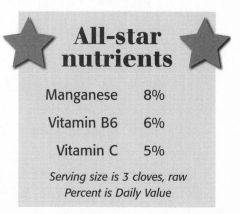

All-star nutrients

Manganese	8%
Vitamin B6	6%
Vitamin C	5%

Serving size is 3 cloves, raw
Percent is Daily Value

■ Studies show that blood-thinning garlic may help prevent clots in your bloodstream. That's good news because heart attacks are often caused by a blood clot that blocks the flow of blood to your heart.

■ The vitamin C in garlic may help prevent artery clogs, too. Inside your blood vessels, harmful molecules called free radicals can attack LDL cholesterol, creating artery-clogging plaque. Over time, that plaque might build up enough to block the blood flow to your heart and cause a heart attack. Yet you can give your arteries the equivalent of a good scrub naturally, and here's how. Vitamin C helps guard your LDL cholesterol against free radical attacks. Plus it may reduce the stiffness of your arteries and keep platelets from clumping together, so plaque is less likely to build up. But garlic can't give you all the vitamin C you need, so get more from foods like sweet peppers and strawberries.

■ Recent research suggests that a slight deficiency in vitamin B6 could raise your odds of coronary artery disease — one of the risk factors for a heart attack. Eating more garlic can help you shore up the B6 levels in your diet. Increase your B6 even more by mixing garlic into other foods containing vitamin B6, like marinara sauce or mashed potatoes.

Studies suggest garlic may also improve high blood pressure, hardening of the arteries, and more, but further research is needed to know for sure. Meanwhile, keep enjoying garlic, and stay tuned for the latest developments.

■ ■ ■ ■ ■ Boost the benefits ■ ■ ■ ■ ■

Cooking can reduce garlic's benefits, but you can get some of them back. Research shows that crushing garlic before you cook it helps retain more health-promoting allicin and other compounds that help keep your blood from clotting. For even better results, let the garlic stand for 10 to 15 minutes after crushing, and then cook it.

Find a treasure "clove" of cancer protection. Get a whiff of this. After studying more than 25,000 people in Italy and Switzerland, researchers found that those who ate the most garlic cut their risk of five different kinds of cancer. In other words, adding more garlic to your diet may help prevent cancer of the mouth, esophagus, larynx, kidney, and colon. Garlic contains compounds that may prevent damage to your DNA, and that could help stop cancer before its starts. So aim for more "clove" encounters, and see what garlic can do for you.

Breathe easier with garlic's help. Asthma, emphysema, and chronic bronchitis can make breathing difficult, but you can take steps to prevent these problems. Research shows that people who get the least vitamin C and manganese are more likely to develop breathing problems associated with asthma. Another study found that diets rich in vitamin C might protect against emphysema and chronic bronchitis. Fortunately, garlic can help you add a little more vitamin C and manganese to your diet at the same time. Sautéing garlic in oil may help even more because it produces vinyldithiins, compounds that help open up your air passageways.

If breathing problems are part of your life, it certainly can't hurt to eat more garlic. But for best results, increase your manganese and vitamin C from other sources as well, like pineapples, citrus fruits, okra, sweet peppers, and rice.

■ ■ ■ ■ *Cook's corner* ■ ■ ■ ■

Pick a better bulb. Choose fresh garlic with dry skin and firm, plump bulbs. Avoid soft, spongy, or shriveled cloves or garlic from the refrigerated produce section. Moisture spoils garlic.

Save the flavor. Store unpeeled garlic heads in a dark, dry, cool place for up to two months. If you refrigerate garlic, use it within three days.

Clobber your cloves. Before peeling garlic, push down on a single clove with the flat side of a broad knife, or whack several cloves with the bottom of a skillet. You can then remove the skin with ease. That also crushes the garlic, which helps preserve the nutrients when cooked.

Leeks

■ ■ ■ ■ ■ ■ ■ ■ ■

Unsung hero packs surprising punch

The protective powers of leeks have been famous for centuries. The Roman Emperor Nero ate leeks daily to protect his singing voice. A more modern superstition claims that leeks also shelter you from lightning. And thanks to their high content of the mineral manganese, leeks also help defend against osteoporosis and asthma.

To find them in your supermarket, hunt for a kind of oversized green onion with almost no bulb. Their dark green flat leaves top a stem that shades from green into white. These stems are edible. Their flavor is onion-like, but delightfully milder and sweeter. Thin baby leeks are even smaller, sweeter, and more tender. You may also find Chinese leeks and wild leeks, also known as ramps. They have a stronger taste.

Iron shields against Alzheimer's danger. Your risk of Alzheimer's may be higher if you

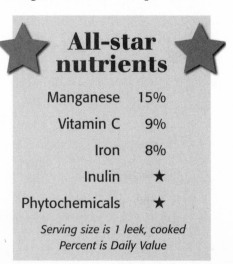

All-star nutrients	
Manganese	15%
Vitamin C	9%
Iron	8%
Inulin	★
Phytochemicals	★

Serving size is 1 leek, cooked
Percent is Daily Value

don't get enough iron. New research shows that even mild iron deficiency can affect a woman's ability to process and use information quickly. What's more, earlier studies suggest missing iron may be one of the factors that causes brain cells to age and die.

Although more research on iron and Alzheimer's risk is needed, the fact remains that older adults are more likely to be iron deficient. By adding leeks and other iron-rich foods to your diet, you can start getting more of this important mineral right away. Just remember to talk with your doctor first if you take iron supplements or a multivitamin containing iron. An overload of iron can suppress your immune system and possibly raise your risk of cancer. Play it safe and get your iron from food unless your doctor recommends otherwise.

■ ■ ■ ■ ■ Boost the benefits ■ ■ ■ ■ ■

To sneak more leeks into your diet, slip chopped leeks into stir fries, casseroles, pasta sauces, or soups. Or sauté your leeks and stir into mashed potatoes.

Surprise nutrient may help diabetes. Inulin may turn out to be the best little nutrient you've never heard of, especially if you have type 2 diabetes. Inulin is a sweet soluble fiber that you naturally get from leeks. But what makes inulin exciting is this — scientists have found evidence it may help lower your blood sugar.

Leeks are a good source of this soluble fiber, which may also help protect against colon cancer, breast cancer, diarrhea, infectious bowel diseases, and maybe even high cholesterol. So don't just add more leeks to your diet. You'll get extra inulin from onions, bananas, garlic, and asparagus, too.

Leeks lock out mouth cancer and more. Fascinating new research from Harvard has made an unlikely discovery. Vitamin C from foods helps prevent cancer of the mouth, but vitamin C from supplements does not. The researchers suspect vitamin C may not be the only nutrient in foods that foils cancer.

And in the case of leeks, they'd almost surely be right. Leeks contain some of the same powerful cancer-fighting phytochemicals that garlic is famous for. Take diallyl sulfide (DAS), for example. DAS may block the dangerous enzymes that turn harmless substances into compounds that help trigger cancer. DAS may also encourage existing cancer cells to die. Leeks may not contain as much DAS as garlic, but they still help armor your body against several kinds of cancer. Even better, leeks won't give you a bad case of "garlic breath" after you eat them.

On top of that, leeks also contain another cancer-fighting phyto-chemical — kaempferol. Kaempferol is a nutritious yellow pigment that tints foods and flowers. It may also help keep you healthy. In a study of more than 60,000 women, those who had the highest intake of kaempferol had 40 percent less risk of ovarian cancer than women with the lowest intake. If you'd like to get extra helpings of kaempferol, enjoy more broccoli, tea, onions, blueberries, kale, and spinach.

■ ■ ■ ■ *Cook's corner* ■ ■ ■ ■

Look for leeks with the largest portion of white and light green. Avoid any that have yellowing, withering, rounded bottoms, or lack crispness.

Store leeks — untrimmed and washed — by wrapping them in damp paper towels and keeping them in the fridge crisper drawer for up to a week.

Trim off the dark green stalks and the rootlets. Slit the remaining portion lengthwise. Hold the resulting layers apart and wash them under cold, running water. Strip off the outermost layer before eating or cooking.

Make old cuisine new again. Use leeks in any recipe you'd use onions or asparagus.

Portabella mushrooms

■■■■■■■■■■■■■■■■■■■■■■

Down-to-earth food builds up your health

Thousands of years ago, people believed mushrooms were magical plants created by bolts of lightning. And, although mushrooms are considered a fungus, they were prized by the nobles of ancient societies, and lower classes were forbidden to eat them.

But that restriction simply couldn't last. Mushroom spores multiply like crazy, so "shrooms" have been actively farmed in caves and gathered from forests for several centuries. And today, names like shiitake, maitake, white button, and portabella are becoming easier to find in markets, menus, and home cooking. You can even order the flat tops or "caps" of grilled portabellas in a scrumptious sandwich in some restaurants. Just remember, picking mushrooms outdoors is dangerous because many are poisonous, so play it safe and pick yours at the supermarket.

Eat mushrooms to your heart's delight. Portabellas serve up two vital nutrients that may help you escape heart attacks and strokes.

Riboflavin. It's not known as a heart-smart star, but don't be fooled. It may protect your heart from behind the scenes — and here's how. Experts believe high blood levels of the amino

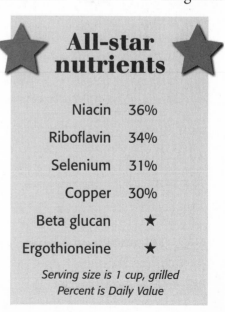

All-star nutrients

Niacin	36%
Riboflavin	34%
Selenium	31%
Copper	30%
Beta glucan	★
Ergothioneine	★

Serving size is 1 cup, grilled
Percent is Daily Value

acid homocysteine can damage and narrow your arteries, which may increase your risk of heart attacks and strokes. Vitamins B6, B12, and folate help lower homocysteine levels, and riboflavin appears to help these vitamins do their job.

Recent studies confirmed that B vitamins lowered homocysteine, but surprisingly, those lower levels did not result in fewer heart problems. Researchers now think homocysteine may simply be a marker for heart disease, not a cause. They no longer recommend supplementing with high doses of B vitamins to protect your heart, but believe a diet rich in these vitamins may provide some benefit.

Beta glucan. Portabellas may also help your heart by lowering your cholesterol levels. They contain a high amount of beta glucan, a soluble fiber that is particularly good at sweeping cholesterol out of your body. Oats are famous for their beta glucan content, but portabellas are a delicious way to help you add the extra servings recommended by the Food and Drug Administration.

■ ■ ■ ■ ■ **Boost the benefits** ■ ■ ■ ■ ■

Don't be afraid to try an exotic mushroom like the shiitake. This little beauty has even more of the antioxidant ergothioneine than portabella mushrooms, plus it has an unusually high amount of vitamin D. Just 3.5 ounces of dried shiitakes give you 1,600 IU of vitamin D — four times what you need in one day. Scientists have discovered that vitamin D helps your body in many ways besides building your bones, and most people don't get enough. Try shiitakes and you'll enjoy a tantalizing, smoky flavor that will give your dishes a boost in taste as well as nutrition.

Cut cancer risk with "cave cuisine." Portabellas may not look like cancer-fighters, but these cave dwellers deliver four hard-hitting nutrients to help keep you cancer free.

Try a variety for better health

Portabellas aren't the only mushrooms that can help you stay healthy.

Eating more white button mushrooms may help boost your immunity and build bonus protection against cancer and viruses, a new animal study suggests. Meanwhile, other animal and lab studies hint that just under a cup a day could help control estrogen and prevent breast cancer.

A small human study suggests that eating a few fresh or dried shiitake mushrooms every day may help lower cholesterol by up to 12 percent — thanks to a mushroom nutrient called eritadenine.

Tests of an extract of another shiitake nutrient — lentinan — reveal exciting news. Not only is lentinan a potentially powerful immune booster, but it also shows promise against cancer.

Portabellas give you plenty of niacin (vitamin B3) as well as tremendous antioxidant power from a nutrient called ergothioneine. According to a European study, eating more niacin and antioxidants could cut your risk of deadly esophageal cancer, mouth cancer, and throat cancer by up to 40 percent.

Several studies also suggest extra vitamin D could help protect you from breast cancer, colon cancer, and more. Mushrooms are the only non-animal source of vitamin D, so they're a good place to start.

As if that weren't enough, portabellas also deliver a blast of selenium. Research suggests people who don't get enough selenium have a higher risk for several kinds of cancer. What's more, men may be in more danger than women because of their risk for prostate cancer. Fortunately, eating selenium-rich foods like portabellas may cut your cancer chances and help keep you safe.

Smart way to fortify your immune system. Consume more 'shrooms, and you could avoid getting sick. That's because portabellas deliver infection-fighting copper and health-promoting ergothioneine.

Although you don't need much copper from foods, you don't want to come up short either. Studies show that copper deficiency may keep your immune system from working properly, and animal studies suggest you'll be more vulnerable to infections if you don't get enough.

Shade-loving mushrooms are also a leading source of ergothioneine and other mighty antioxidants. Believe it or not, mushrooms boast more antioxidant power than tomatoes, carrots, or green peppers, giving you a better chance of dodging chronic diseases like Alzheimer's, cancer, and hardening of the arteries.

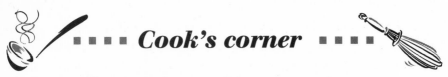

▪ ▪ ▪ ▪ *Cook's corner* ▪ ▪ ▪ ▪

- Choose mushrooms with spongy, supple tops. Avoid mushrooms with black spots or any that look shriveled, discolored, wet, or slippery.

- Store unwashed mushrooms in a paper bag or wrapped in paper towels for up to three days. Dried mushrooms may keep for several months.

- To clean mushrooms, just wipe them with a damp paper towel. Never soak or dunk fresh mushrooms in water. You can rinse them quickly if they're very dirty. To plump up dried mushrooms, soak them in warm water for about 20-30 minutes.

Romaine lettuce

■ ■

Nutritional superstar hides in a humble leaf

Ancient Romans once ate lettuce as a dessert. But after a romaine lettuce "prescription" helped Augustus Caesar recover from serious illness, he put up a statue to honor romaine for its healing powers instead.

Perhaps he had the right idea. Romaine lettuce is far more nutritious than the iceberg lettuce most people eat. For example, romaine lettuce has almost three times as much vitamin K as iceberg. That extra vitamin K may help you avoid disabling problems like osteoporosis and osteoarthritis.

Romaine is also loaded with other nutrients, so try it anywhere you'd normally use iceberg lettuce. You may be pleasantly surprised at how it can make a good dish even better. And don't forget romaine lettuce is a must-have for a truly tantalizing Caesar salad.

Bite into a better asthma fighter. Turn over a new leaf and you might avoid asthma symptoms. A study of French women revealed that those who ate the most lettuce, spinach, and other leafy greens were 22 percent less likely to have asthma. Vitamin A may be the reason why. Not only is it found in both lettuce and spinach, but this vital vitamin also defends your immune system and protects the lining of your lungs. Even better, if you choose romaine instead of the usual iceberg lettuce, you'll nab almost eight times as much vitamin A.

But vitamin A isn't the only asthma-fighting nutrient in luscious romaine lettuce. This high-powered green also delivers healthy amounts of vitamin C and manganese. A British

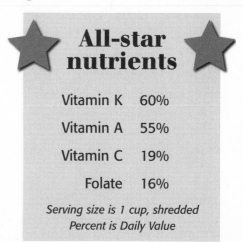

All-star nutrients

Vitamin K	60%
Vitamin A	55%
Vitamin C	19%
Folate	16%

Serving size is 1 cup, shredded
Percent is Daily Value

study found that people who got more vitamin C and manganese were less likely to develop asthma symptoms.

As with vitamin A, choosing romaine lettuce over iceberg can help. Romaine lettuce has six times as much vitamin C as iceberg lettuce. To add extra manganese, top your romaine lettuce with blackberries or chopped pineapple.

■ ■ ■ ■ ■ Boost the benefits ■ ■ ■ ■ ■

Order the chef salad at one chain restaurant and you'll get twice as many calories and fat grams as a fast food double cheeseburger. So when you belly up to the salad bar, use these tips to avoid health sabotage and assemble a deliciously healthy salad instead.

- Substitute Parmesan cheese for cheddar or feta cheese.
- Switch from bacon bits to sunflower seeds.
- Choose romaine or other greens over iceberg lettuce.
- Substitute low-fat or nonfat dressings for full-fat versions.
- Emphasize foods like chickpeas, carrots, beets, mushrooms, broccoli, cauliflower, and tomatoes.
- Avoid croutons, Chinese noodles, and anything containing mayonnaise or oil.

Bowl over Alzheimer's risk with salad. You might not think of romaine lettuce as "brain food," but research from Harvard Medical School suggests it can be. In a study of over 13,000 women, those who ate the most romaine lettuce and other leafy greens experienced less decline in mental ability than women who ate the least.

The researchers think the honors go to one of romaine's powerful nutrients — folate, a B vitamin that has lowered the risk of Alzheimer's disease in other studies. Folate suppresses the blood levels of the amino acid homocysteine. That's important because lab and animal studies suggest high homocysteine levels may have toxic effects on your brain cells. It may also cause your risk of Alzheimer's to skyrocket.

Also, be sure to get enough vitamin B12 along with your folate or you might raise your risk of damaged brain cells. Older adults are more likely to be deficient in vitamin B12. Your doctor can check you for a B12 deficiency. Meanwhile, get more B12 from foods like fish, chicken, eggs, lean red meat, and low-fat milk and cheese. For extra folate, enjoy plenty of romaine lettuce and try foods like rice, lentils, and fortified cereal.

Cut hunger pangs and shed pounds. Eating lettuce might help you lose weight without feeling hungry all the time. Here's why. Low-calorie foods can make you feel full if they also have a high water content. And any type of lettuce you can think of is at least 90 percent water.

This may sound like just another shaky diet claim, but science suggests it can really work. One research study found that drinking water before a meal reduces the total number of calories older adults chose to eat. The water also helped them feel more full. Another study found that a big, low-calorie salad before a meal can have similar calorie-slashing effects on the entire meal. So if you're struggling to lose weight, why not try a low calorie "appetizer" salad. You have nothing to lose but pounds and inches.

Pick higher-powered lettuce to stay well

The lettuce you choose for your salad can make a big difference in how much nutrition you get. Just look at the numbers for a cup of each kind of lettuce to see for yourself. Keep in mind the percent is the Daily Value.

Nutrient	Iceberg	Romaine	Boston/ Bibb	Red leaf	Radicchio	Arugula
Vitamin A	7%	55%	36%	42%	0%	10%
Vitamin C	3%	19%	3%	2%	5%	4%
Vitamin K	22%	60%	70%	49%	128%	28%
Folate	5%	16%	10%	3%	6%	4%
Manganese	4%	4%	5%	3%	3%	4%
Potassium	3%	3%	4%	1%	3%	2%
Iron	2%	3%	4%	2%	1%	2%

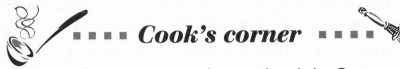

Cook's corner

Look for very green, crisp leaves with no holes. Outer leaves should curl away from the inner leaves. Avoid large, milky ribs and heads with hints of rust.

Wash thoroughly and drain or blot dry. Store unwashed romaine lettuce in a bag in the refrigerator for up to one week. Keep well away from fruits like apples, bananas, and pears.

Pop your lettuce into the freezer for two minutes before eating or serving if it seems a bit less crisp than you like.

Use in Caesar salads, regular salads, and sandwiches. Lettuce leaves are also a wrapper's delight, so curl them around veggies or any combination of sandwich ingredients.

Rutabagas

Supercharge your health with a curious veggie

You might not think of rutabagas as holiday food, but that's exactly what they are in Scotland. In fact, rutabagas are the "neeps" of "tatties and neeps," a dish traditionally served on Scotland's Burns Night holiday.

You might also be surprised to learn rutabagas are cancer-fighting members of the cabbage family. This little-known root vegetable is a cross between a cabbage and a turnip. As a result, the rutabaga looks like a pale version of an extra-large turnip. But don't be fooled. Rutabagas taste sweeter than turnips, so plan accordingly when you use them in cooking.

Win against diverticulosis with fiber. You may not think of rutabagas when people talk about "bulking up," but you will now. Rutabagas have plenty of fiber to help you escape diverticulosis — or keep it from becoming painful diverticulitis. Here's how it works.

Constipation causes high pressure in your colon that can create weak spots or pouches called diverticula. That's where fiber comes in. It helps ease the pressure by softening and bulking up your stools, which keeps things moving along. That may keep new diverticula from forming or even prevent them in the first place. In fact, one study found that men who ate the most fiber were 42 percent less likely to develop diverticulosis compared with men who ate little fiber.

So if you're over age 60, consider adding more of two elements to your diet. First, add more fiber to your meals. Rutabagas are a good place to start. Other good choices include beans, dates, and whole grain breakfast cereals. Second, drink lots of water and add fiber gradually so you'll avoid unpleasant side effects, like gas and bloating. Take these steps and you'll help prevent diverticulosis or stop it from getting worse.

Eat rutabagas to prevent breathing problems. Nearly 10 million people are diagnosed with emphysema or chronic bronchitis every year. If you want to keep your lungs healthy, enjoying more rutabagas may help.

Research from the University of Nottingham in England suggests people who get more vitamin C and magnesium from their diets have healthier lungs. What's more, people who eat more vitamin C lose significantly less lung function over the long haul. That may lower your risk of breathing problems from emphysema and chronic bronchitis.

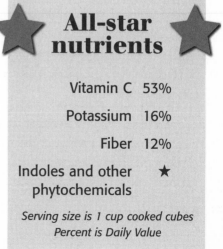

All-star nutrients

Vitamin C 53%

Potassium 16%

Fiber 12%

Indoles and other phytochemicals ★

Serving size is 1 cup cooked cubes
Percent is Daily Value

101

To get more vitamin C and magnesium, start with rutabagas. Be sure to munch other top vitamin C sources like sweet peppers, oranges, strawberries, broccoli, and kiwi, too. For extra magnesium, consider black beans, halibut, spinach, and white beans.

Some evidence indicates that people deficient in nutrients like potassium and vitamin C also have a higher risk of losing lung function and having breathing difficulties. Rutabagas can help you avoid a deficiency in either nutrient. You'll add extra potassium if you enjoy your rutabagas with a baked potato, lima beans, or winter squash or have a banana or some dates for dessert.

■ ■ ■ ■ ■ **Boost the benefits** ■ ■ ■ ■ ■

Sneak cubed rutabaga into soups, casseroles, or stews, or slip chopped or sliced raw rutabaga into salads. Rutabagas can also be mashed after cooking and then mixed into mashed potatoes. If these tricks don't convert your rutabaga-haters or just don't taste good to you, try steaming or baking your rutabagas and then mash them with butter and cinnamon.

Reduce your risk of cancer. These days, it seems nearly everything causes cancer. You probably feel as if your body needs a 24-hour watch team to constantly seek out and stop potential threats. Fortunately, that's exactly what rutabagas do. These veggies come equipped with a SWAT team of powerful cancer-fighting phytochemicals and here's what they can do for you.

- *Sulforaphane.* The average antioxidant stops working the moment it neutralizes a cancer-causing molecule in your body, but the phytochemical sulforaphane triggers a days-long defense from your body's phase-2 detoxification enzymes. These enzymes spur your immune system to hunt down cancer-causing compounds and remove them from your body.

- *Indole-3-carbinol.* Another phytochemical, called indole-3-carbinol (I3C), also raises your count of phase 2 enzymes. But I3C also helps prevent your body's estrogen from becoming a cancer-causing compound. Some animal studies suggest I3C might raise your cancer risk if it comes from supplements, so get your I3C from tasty foods, like rutabagas.

- *Dithiolethione.* The phytochemical dithiolthione may be tough to pronounce, but it's tough on cancer, too. Not only can it help destroy cancer-causing compounds, it may also help stop the growth of cancer cells. Plus, new animal research suggests dithiolthione cranks up your immune system, so you fight cancer even more effectively.

- *Isothiocyanates.* A group of phytochemicals called isothiocyanates help boost your body's antioxidant count. What's more, both I3C and isothiocyanates help destroy cancer-causing compounds you may get from foods and other sources. Unfortunately, some cancer-causers may still sneak into your body. Once there, they can damage your DNA, which can turn normal cells into cancer. But indoles and isothiocyanates lay in wait to help prevent DNA damage and keep you safe.

When to avoid rutabagas

Rutabagas are not safe for everyone. If you have diabetes, rutabagas could raise your blood sugar, thanks to their high ranking on the glycemic index. If you have thyroid problems, be aware that rutabagas contain goitrogens, natural chemicals that interfere with your thyroid hormones and iodine levels. Rutabagas are also high in the oxalates that could trigger kidney stones, and they may contain other kidney-troubling compounds.

If you have thyroid problems, kidney problems, or diabetes, talk to your doctor before eating rutabagas. She can tell you whether you must avoid rutabagas or merely limit the amounts you eat.

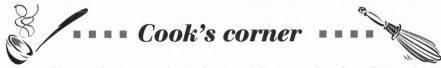

■ ■ ■ ■ *Cook's corner* ■ ■ ■ ■

Choose firm, smooth rutabagas without cracks, shriveling, and soft spots. They should feel heavy for their size and be nearly free of roots at the base.

Before cooking, scrub the rutabaga under cool running water. Cut off its top and bottom. Put the cut side down and split into quarters. Rutabagas are often coated in wax to keep them from drying out. So use a paring knife to peel the skin from rutabaga quarters before cooking or eating.

Store unwashed rutabagas in a plastic bag in the refrigerator for up to 2 weeks.

Spinach
■ ■ ■ ■ ■ ■ ■ ■ ■ ■ ■ ■

Pack a nutrient-rich punch with a popular green

Spinach was never delivered by magic carpets, but this nutritious veggie probably did get its start in ancient Persia. It has since become popular everywhere from China to the United States. Arabs even call spinach the prince of vegetables.

They may have the right idea. Spinach is loaded with nutrients including vitamin A, vitamin K, manganese, folate, vitamin C, and the sight-saving phytochemicals lutein and zeaxanthin. This leafy green also contains plenty of iron and calcium, but the oxalates in spinach prevent you from absorbing much of either one. Seek calcium and iron from other foods, like cereals, dairy products, and clams.

Also, be aware that certain substances in spinach aren't safe for everyone. If you have kidney stones, thyroid problems, or if you take a blood thinner, like warfarin, ask your doctor for advice.

Eat your greens to prevent a stroke. Make leafy greens, like spinach, your new best friends. Just one serving per day lowers your risk of heart disease and stroke by 11 percent, researchers report. What's more, these green machines may even protect you if you ever have a stroke. An animal study found that rats that ate spinach-enriched diets experienced less damage from a stroke than rats that ate no spinach.

Researchers suspect spinach may help protect you in several ways. It contains antioxidants and anti-inflammatory compounds that may protect your brain from damage. It's also high in folate, a valuable B vitamin you need every day.

A recent study discovered that folate supplements could help lower your risk of stroke. But one expert warns that supplements may raise the risk of heart disease in some people. Don't try supplements unless your doctor approves. Instead, stick with delicious folate-loaded foods, like spinach, rice, and cereals.

Stop varicose veins before they start. Even rock stars aren't immune to varicose veins. One famous rocker recently admitted to struggling with his unsightly veins for years before treating them with surgery and injections. But if you'd rather avoid scalpels and needles, your best bet is to prevent varicose veins in the first place.

Fortunately, a new test tube study suggests vitamin K supplements may help you avoid varicose veins. Researchers think vitamin K may short-circuit a process that causes such veins. More research is needed, but you can start eating more vitamin K-rich foods now. A cup of crisp, raw spinach supplies you with 181 percent of the recommended

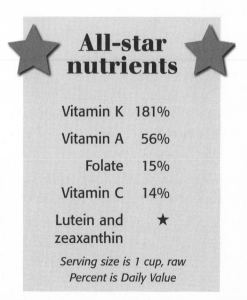

All-star nutrients

Vitamin K	181%
Vitamin A	56%
Folate	15%
Vitamin C	14%
Lutein and zeaxanthin	★

Serving size is 1 cup, raw
Percent is Daily Value

daily value for vitamin K. Other good sources include kale, collards, and turnip greens. Just remember, if you take warfarin or other blood thinners, don't eat foods high in vitamin K unless your doctor says it's safe.

■ ■ ■ ■ ■ **Boost the benefits** ■ ■ ■ ■ ■

To get the most nutrition from your spinach, use it quickly. Fresh spinach can lose as much as 54 percent of its carotenoids and 47 percent of its folate during the first four days of storage if left unrefrigerated. But after eight days, even refrigerated spinach loses 56 percent of carotenoids and 47 percent of folate. If you can't use it quickly, buy frozen spinach.

And if you're concerned about food poisoning, a Purdue University expert recommends bagged spinach. It's less likely to become contaminated during transport or at the super-market. Choose bags labeled "triple washed." For even more protection, cook your spinach.

Gang up on colon cancer danger. Here's good news if you or some-one you love adores red meat. Spinach can help reduce the colon cancer risk from meat.

A Dutch animal study discovered that spinach and its chlorophyll — the green pigment of plants — can help keep the heme in red meat from making cancer-causing changes in your colon. This doesn't mean you can go hog wild eating red meat, but you may be safer if you also eat more spinach. Besides, spinach is loaded with several nutrients that help you resist cancer.

Beta carotene is converted into vitamin A in your body, but both beta carotene and vitamin A are cancer-fighting antioxidants. What's more, diets rich in beta carotene and other carotenoids slash the risk of colon cancer.

The vitamin C in spinach helps fight cancer-causing nitrosamines in meats and other foods you eat. Research shows that a vitamin-C shortfall raises your risk of cancer, but eating high amounts of this vitamin lowers that risk.

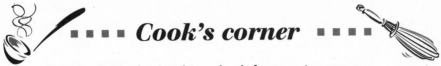

Cook's corner

Squeeze bagged spinach to check for a springy texture.

Store fresh, unwashed spinach in a plastic bag in your refrigerator crisper for up to four days. Don't store cooked spinach.

Trim off roots and separate the leaves. Drop the spinach into a large bowl of room-temperature water. Stir to dislodge dirt. Replace the dirty water with clean water and swirl again. Repeat until no dirt appears in the water. Shake raw spinach dry in a colander before adding to salads or sandwiches.

Cut off thick stems before cooking. Speedy cooking methods for spinach include sautéing, steaming, and microwaving.

Spring onions

Delicate taste offers tough protection

If the taste of regular, round onions has always been too harsh for you, try spring onions. They have a milder flavor, but still enough bite to be delicious. Like most onions, spring onions got their start in Asia. But, unlike other onions, spring onions aren't round at all. Instead, their green, leafy tops rise out of a nearly straight white base. Both the base and the top are edible so be sure to look for these zippy veggies at your supermarket. Just remember to read the labels, too. Spring onions may be tagged "green onions" or "scallions."

Chop arthritis pain with onions. Scientists say osteoarthritis pain has been around so long that even the dinosaurs experienced it. But that doesn't mean you have to wait a million years to feel better. Amazing nutrients found in onions may start helping you much sooner.

In spite of their reputation for a taste "with a kick," onions contain anti-inflammatories — compounds like vitamin C, quercetin, and isothiocyanates — that squelch inflammation-triggering enzymes and help prevent pain and swelling. In fact, research shows that a high vitamin-C intake can help reduce knee pain and slow the progress of osteoarthritis.

The vitamin K in onions may also help keep your symptoms from getting worse. One study found that people with low blood levels of vitamin K were more prone to bone spurs and other signs of osteoarthritis in their knees and hands. Fortunately, higher vitamin K levels meant fewer symptoms. Just remember, if you take warfarin or another blood-thinning drug, talk to your doctor before eating foods high in vitamin K.

Guard against lung disease. Even if you've never smoked, you could still be in danger of emphysema or chronic bronchitis. Cooks, miners, food workers who work in tight quarters, and anyone regularly exposed to dust, smoke, or other pollutants are at higher risk. But onions can help protect you — and here's why.

Onions are a good source of beta carotene. Nonsmokers who eat the most foods rich in beta carotene have less loss of lung function than people who eat less, research shows. That's good news because a speedier loss of lung function may be an early sign of emphysema or chronic bronchitis. So eat a few more onions and other foods with beta carotene — like carrots. They might help you breathe easier for a long time.

Flavorful way to fend off cancer. Eating more onions could help you avoid five kinds of cancer — including one of the

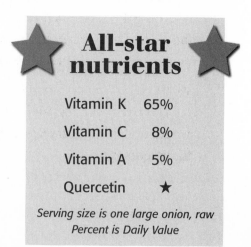

All-star nutrients

Vitamin K	65%
Vitamin C	8%
Vitamin A	5%
Quercetin	★

Serving size is one large onion, raw
Percent is Daily Value

most dangerous kinds. A European study found that people who ate the most onions cut their risk of colon cancer, ovarian cancer, oral cancer, cancer of the larynx, and the very deadly cancer of the esophagus.

But spring onions may not be your best means of preventing cancer. Cornell University tests showed that sweet onions aren't as effective at fighting cancer as stronger-tasting round onions. The researchers didn't test spring onions, so nobody knows whether they carry more or less cancer-fighting power than their sweeter cousins. But don't abandon spring onions. Studies suggest their beta carotene can help prevent stomach cancer.

Onions offer other benefits, too. Early research suggests an onion compound called allyl propyl disulphide can fight high blood sugar. Spring onions may also help prevent blood clots that cause heart attacks. In fact, eating the quercetin found in onions, tea, and apples has been linked to a lower heart attack risk — and your body may absorb more quercetin from onions than from other sources. As if that weren't enough, onions contain powerful compounds that kill some of the harmful bacteria that can make you sick.

■ ■ ■ ■ ■ Boost the benefits ■ ■ ■ ■ ■

Although spring onions are a good start on your daily intake of vitamins C and A, you'll need other foods to help you reach the recommended amounts. Rich vitamin C foods include strawberries, cranberry juice cocktail, papaya, orange juice from concentrate, and brussels sprouts.

Your body can make vitamin A from beta carotene, so eat champion beta carotene sources like baked sweet potatoes, canned pumpkin, collards, cooked carrots, and turnip greens.

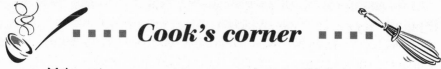

Cook's corner

Make onion preparation easy on the eyes. Chill the onion before chopping it — and use your sharpest knife.

Store unwashed spring onions in a plastic bag in your refrigerator for up to five days. Store regular onions in a burlap bag in a place that is cool, dark, and dry. But don't store onions with potatoes. The moisture from potatoes makes onions spoil faster.

The best spring onions are less than a half inch thick — or smaller than the width of a dime.

Sweet green peppers

Silence health risks with a 'bell'

Just one sweet green bell pepper gives you more vitamin C than a whole orange — 35 percent more. These bell-shaped peppers are also a rich source of vitamin K, a mighty nutrient that might help you avoid disabling osteoporosis and osteoarthritis. But that's just the beginning.

Green bell peppers are the teenagers of the pepper world. If they stay on the pepper plant long enough, they turn into vibrant red bell peppers, which are even sweeter. Bell peppers also come in orange, yellow, and purple.

But no matter which peck of peppers you pick, you'll find many tempting ways to eat them. Snack on fresh, raw peppers or add them to salads. Fill a whole, lightly steamed pepper with rice pilaf or add chopped peppers to stir fries, stews, or Cajun foods. You can even roast red peppers to add tangy flavor to pasta.

Save your teeth with pepper power. The bright colors of bell peppers don't just make your dishes more vibrant. They also deliver two nutrients that protect your teeth — vitamin B6 and vitamin C.

A small Japanese study discovered that people who get more of a particular group of nutrients may be less likely to lose their teeth. Vitamin B6 was one of these crucial nutrients, and bell peppers help you get more. Other teeth protectors include vitamin B1, niacin, vitamin D, and protein. So why not serve up some salmon on a bed of brown rice, chopped bell peppers, and tomatoes. You'll get a delicious meal plus nutrients your teeth will love.

This dish also delivers vitamin C, and many gum disease specialists recommend vitamin C for healthy gums. Studies suggest this vitamin may help prevent the gum diseases that can lead to tooth loss. Vitamin C's ability to repair the connective tissue in gums may help protect your teeth, too.

Add pepper protection to your anti-arthritis artillery. People who have recently developed inflammatory polyarthritis —inflammation of more than one joint — may be more likely to get rheumatoid arthritis, according to British researchers. Fortunately, eating bell peppers might help. A University of Manchester study found that people who got the least vitamin C from their diets had three times as much risk of inflammatory polyarthritis. While you can get vitamin C from papaya, strawberries, and cranberry juice cocktail, don't let that tempt you to bypass peppers. Not only are

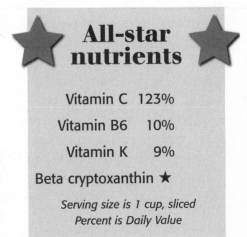

All-star nutrients

Vitamin C   123%

Vitamin B6   10%

Vitamin K   9%

Beta cryptoxanthin ★

Serving size is 1 cup, sliced
Percent is Daily Value

green and red peppers a leading source of vitamin C, but they may also have something extra to offer.

Research suggests that people who get the most beta cryptoxanthin from food are also at less risk of inflammatory polyarthritis. Green peppers supply some of this valuable phytochemical, but red peppers deliver so much that few foods can give you more. So sneak red bell peppers into your meals whenever you can. For extra vitamin C and beta cryptoxanthin, enjoy oranges and orange juice, too.

■ ■ ■ ■ ■ Boost the benefits ■ ■ ■ ■ ■

Compared with green peppers, raw red peppers have eight times as much vitamin A, seven times as much beta carotene, 70 times as much beta cryptoxanthin, and 28 percent more vitamin C. When raw, red peppers also give you lycopene. Green peppers don't. But raw, green peppers still deliver six times as much lutein and zeaxanthin as raw, red peppers, so eat them, too.

To get the most vitamin A, alpha carotene, beta carotene, and beta cryptoxanthin from peppers, eat them with olive oil or another healthy fat.

Eat these "sweets" to beat lung cancer risk. If you're worried about your lung cancer risk, grab a sweet bell pepper and start munching. Research suggests a passion for these peppers could help you escape lung cancer. The secret may be their vitamin C. A 25-year research study found that men who got more than 83 milligrams (mg) of vitamin C from food every day had a lower risk of lung cancer than men who got less. You can get 80 mg from just two-thirds of a cup of chopped green bell peppers. That ought to be enough to make these peppers your dinner bells, but there's more. A research review found that beta cryptoxanthin also helps lower lung cancer odds. Red peppers are rich in this phytochemical, so be sure to eat red peppers as well as green.

■ ■ ■ ■ ■ *Cook's corner* **■ ■ ■ ■ ■**

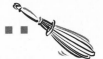

■ If green bell peppers cause burping and indigestion, peel the skin.

■ Keep unwashed peppers in a plastic bag or the crisper in your refrigerator for up to four days, but remember that red peppers will spoil before green ones.

■ Before cutting a bell pepper, hold it with the bottom end in your palm and whack the stem against the counter to loosen the seed pack inside. Then cut off the stem, slice the pepper in half, and remove the seeds. Slice or chop with the skin side down.

■ Wash unwaxed peppers under running water, but scrub the ones that are waxed.

Sweet potatoes

Uncover nature's sweet rewards

Sweet potatoes are the number one food for better health, according to the Center for Science in the Public Interest. And it's no wonder. This tasty tuber is so nutritious that early settlers on the American frontier depended on it to survive. The sweet potato not only gave them vital minerals, like potassium and manganese, but also plenty of nourishing vitamins and phytochemicals to restore weary bodies and spirits.

Sweet potatoes were also key to the diets of Revolutionary War soldiers, Mexico's Aztec Indians, and the Inca Indians of Peru. Any food that keeps so many people going is too important to restrict to Thanksgiving, so enjoy sweet potatoes year round. They're easy to bake, and they make a deliciously healthy side dish to any meal.

Enjoy a diabetes-friendly food. Even if you have diabetes, a sweet potato is one sweet treat you can probably eat. Unlike regular white potatoes, sweet potatoes aren't high on the glycemic index. What's more, they have a naturally sweet taste that grows even sweeter as they're stored or cooked. One bite and you'll be saying, "How sweet it is," like the popular entertainer Jackie Gleason.

On top of that, scientists have linked deficiencies in beta carotene, vitamin E, and vitamin B6 to higher blood sugar levels. Although sweet potatoes only supply a little vitamin E, they're a good source of vitamin B6, and they're brimming with beta carotene. That extra nutrition may also help control your blood sugar.

The down side to sweet potatoes is that they're not as low in calories as a plain baked white potato. But you can still enjoy these healthy sweets if you remember two rules. First, don't load a sweet potato with high-fat toppings or high-calorie ingredients. Second, subtract a few calories from another part of your day so your total calorie count won't rise.

Meanwhile, keep an ear to the ground because a white sweet potato from the Japanese mountains may soon help people with diabetes even more. An extract from this sweet potato is used to make a food additive called caiapo. Researchers say three months of caiapo helped lower both cholesterol and blood sugar in people with type 2 diabetes. So stay tuned for the latest news.

Arm your body with natural ulcer fighters. Not only can

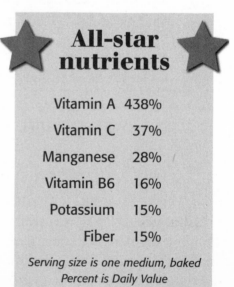

All-star nutrients

Vitamin A	438%
Vitamin C	37%
Manganese	28%
Vitamin B6	16%
Potassium	15%
Fiber	15%

Serving size is one medium, baked
Percent is Daily Value

a fiber-rich diet slash your chances of getting an ulcer, but that same fiber may also help an ulcer heal faster if you already have one. For the most powerful fiber protection, choose delicious produce like sweet potatoes. Their vitamin A makes them even more effective.

Their vitamin C isn't "small potatoes," either. One research study suggested people with low blood levels of vitamin C are more likely to become infected by *H. pylori* — the bacteria known for causing ulcers. Although antibiotics cure 70 to 90 percent of the *H. pylori* ulcers, your best bet is to fight your infection risk before ulcers happen. So beef up your defenses with extra vitamin C, fiber, and vitamin A from produce. Start with good choices like sweet potatoes, turnip greens, raw broccoli, and sweet red peppers.

■ ■ ■ ■ ■ Boost the benefits ■ ■ ■ ■ ■

You can safely eat up to a half cup of sweet potatoes without cooking them, but eating more than that causes gas and may have other effects. On the other hand, cooking your sweet potato helps your body absorb more of its fabulous nutrients.

Instead of combining sweet potatoes with fattening, unhealthy choices like brown sugar, marshmallows, or butter, try cinnamon, olive oil, ginger, pineapple, honey, rosemary, apple juice, orange juice, or nutmeg.

Foil gallstones with this dynamic duo. Alexander the Great may have died from gallstones, today's doctors say. But he might have completely avoided stones if he'd only loaded up on two sweet potato nutrients — fiber and vitamin C.

Gallstones get their start when bile stagnates in your gallbladder. The cholesterol in bile can build up and crystallize into stones. Although bile travels to your intestines whenever you need to digest fats, your body reabsorbs the cholesterol from bile when digesting is done. But if soluble fiber is in your intestines, it absorbs the bile and cholesterol instead, flushing them out of your body. What's more, insoluble fiber speeds food through your body so cholesterol has less opportunity to form in the first place. Perhaps that's why eating lots of fiber has been linked to a drop in gallstone danger.

Vitamin C may lend a hand by breaking down cholesterol so it can't form stones. That would certainly help explain why a higher risk of gallstones is associated with vitamin C deficiency. On top of that, a study found that women with high blood levels of C reduced their risk of gallbladder disease.

Pit this potato against colds and flu. That beautiful blaze of autumn leaf colors may mean cold and flu season is fast approaching, but you can fight back. Delicious, orange-fleshed sweet potatoes have three ingredients to help resist colds and flu — vitamin A, vitamin B6, and vitamin C. In fact, getting more of these nutrients may leave you with nothing to sneeze at.

- The beta carotene in sweet potatoes turns into vitamin A in your body. That vitamin helps you make more antibodies and disease-fighting cells called lymphocytes so your immune system can better defend you against what's "going around."

- A deficiency in vitamin B6 lowers immunity, but getting more B6 helps make your immune system more powerful.

- Don't give up on vitamin C either. Although researchers found that starting 200 milligrams of daily vitamin C during a cold doesn't make the cold shorter or less severe, getting plenty of vitamin C from food is still a good idea. Vitamin C helps block viruses and supports your immune system. Besides, your bacteria-fighting white blood cells need this vitamin, so don't scrimp. Eat plenty of high C foods like sweet potatoes, orange juice, and bell peppers.

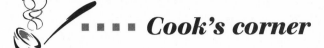

Cook's corner

Don't store raw sweet potatoes in your refrigerator because temperatures below 50 degrees Fahrenheit turn these taters tough and rough-tasting. Instead, find a dark, dry place with good air circulation and temperatures in the 50s. Sweet potatoes will last 10 days under these conditions. You can store cooked sweet potatoes in your refrigerator for up to a week.

Tomatoes

Go red to get into the pink of health

When you eat a tomato, you're actually eating a berry, botanists say. It is classified that way because it is pulpy and contains seeds, not stones. In fact, the first tomatoes growing in western South America were not much bigger than berries.

Years later, the Aztec Indians triggered the tomato's rise to fame by naming it tomatl and growing it in King Montezuma's gardens.

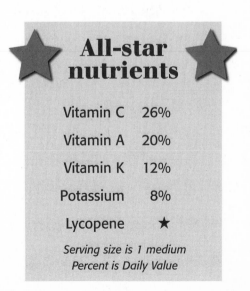

All-star nutrients

Vitamin C	26%
Vitamin A	20%
Vitamin K	12%
Potassium	8%
Lycopene	★

Serving size is 1 medium
Percent is Daily Value

117

That opened the door for Europeans to discover the tomato and introduce it to the rest of the world.

Today, of course, we think of tomatoes as a vegetable. We know these luscious gems are a tasty, healthy treat and great source of potassium, vitamin C, vitamin K, and vitamin A. Red tomatoes are also brimming with lycopene — a phytochemical that is thought to play an important role in preventing disease. Whether raw or cooked, tomatoes add flavor, color, and nutrition to a wide variety of dishes.

■ ■ ■ ■ ■ **Boost the benefits** ■ ■ ■ ■ ■

Cooked tomatoes may deliver more lycopene, but raw tomatoes have more vitamin C, so make both a regular part of your diet. And don't peel them. Unpeeled tomatoes give you more lycopene, beta carotene, kaempferol, and quercetin.

Using plant-sterol spreads like Benecol may cause a 10 to 20 percent drop in your blood levels of the carotenoids alpha carotene, beta carotene, and lycopene, some studies suggest. Add an extra daily serving of carotenoid-rich fruits or veggies to make up the loss.

If spaghetti sauce or other tomato-based foods are too acidic, add chopped carrots. The extra fiber seems to weaken the acidity without affecting flavor — plus you get extra carotenoids.

Harness tomatoes' cancer-fighting power. Lycopene is a powerful antioxidant that experts had touted as a possible way to prevent prostate cancer. Unfortunately, a new study involving 28,000 men found no evidence that lycopene has any effect on prostate cancer. Still, research has shown that tomatoes and their lycopene may help prevent at least four other cancers.

- Nitrosamines from processed meats can form cancer-causing compounds in your digestive tract. Tomatoes come to the rescue with courmaric acid and chlorogenic acid — compounds that block nitrosamines from taking up their cancer-starting ways.

- Pancreatic cancer is the fourth leading cause of cancer among men, and only 5 percent of those diagnosed are still alive five years later. But a Canadian study discovered that men who ate the most lycopene slashed their risk of pancreatic cancer by nearly a third.

- Tomatoes have two ingredients that may help protect against ovarian cancer. Alpha carotene helps prevent this scary cancer after menopause, while lycopene lowers your risk before menopause.

- Similarly, the lycopene in tomatoes may help lower your risk of breast cancer after menopause, while their lutein may help protect you before menopause arrives. Additional phytochemicals called phytoene and phytofluene may also pitch in to show breast cancer who's boss.

So start enjoying more raw tomatoes, pasta sauce, tomato juice, salsa, sun-dried tomatoes, and tomato-based soups. You'll rev up your diet while supplying your body with powerful anti-cancer nutrients.

'Magic' remedy for food poisoning

People once mistakenly thought tomatoes were poisonous. That was proven false, but some foods are genuinely dangerous because bacteria in them can cause food poisoning.

According to an old folk remedy, just two teaspoons of vinegar mixed with water could stop food poisoning before it stops you. If you're worried about something you've eaten, particularly in a foreign country, mix two teaspoons of apple cider vinegar into a tall glass of mineral water, and drink up. If you're lucky, the vinegar will kill the bacteria before trouble starts.

Slice heart attack risk with a golden apple. A medieval Italian botanist labeled the tomato "pomodoro" — meaning golden apple. Although he was probably naming a yellow tomato, it's the bright red varieties that may be as good as gold to your heart.

A study of nearly 40,000 women discovered that tomato-based foods significantly reduced heart disease risk. Tomato sauce and pizza were particularly effective. The potassium in tomatoes may be one reason why. High blood pressure is a key risk factor for heart attacks, but potassium is famous for its power to help control high blood pressure.

Lycopene may lend a hand as well by keeping LDL cholesterol from oxidizing. That oxidation helps plaque build up inside artery walls until blood can't pass through anymore. Studies suggest that tomatoes may help thin your blood so clots are less likely to form and block your arteries.

Tiny dangers like these can add up to big heart problems. Avoid them by eating more tomatoes and tomato-based favorites.

Take a saucy approach to wrinkle prevention. New research suggests many sunscreens may not work as well as previously thought. Some block UV-B rays but not UV-A, yet UV-A can cause the same kinds of skin damage as UV-B. What's more, many people may not apply sunscreen properly or use it frequently enough, so they may not get the SPF protection they're expecting. In other words, you may be at higher risk for sunburn, skin damage, wrinkling, and cancer than you realized. But believe it or not, tomato sauce could help.

Lycopene and other tomato nutrients — like phytofluene and phytoene — may help protect you from sun-caused skin damage. One research study showed that volunteers who regularly drank a tomato extract beverage became less prone to skin reddening after exposure to UV light. While tomatoes and tomato sauces are no substitute for sunscreen or for following sun protection guidelines, eating more tomato treats is a delicious, easy way to help defend your skin.

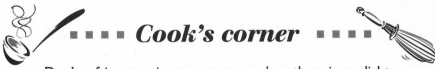

•••• *Cook's corner* ••••

Don't refrigerate ripe tomatoes or place them in sunlight. Refrigerating tomatoes robs them of flavor, and sunlight cuts their vitamin C and makes them ripen unevenly. Instead, store tomatoes stem side down at room temperature. Once they're ripe, use them within two days.

For less splattering, cut tomatoes from stem top to the bottom instead of horizontally.

Before you store pasta sauce in a plastic container, coat it with cooking spray to help prevent staining.

Turnip greens

■ ■

Bank on better health from leafy greens

According to Southern tradition, eating turnip greens on New Year's Day will bring you more green dollar bills all year long. Even if that trick doesn't work, turnip greens can still make you rich in nutrients that help keep you healthy and independent. For example, turnip greens give you a good dose of fiber, vitamin E, folate, calcium, copper, manganese, and beta carotene.

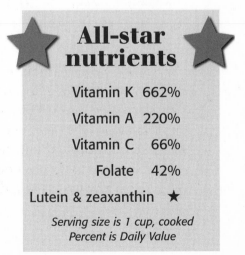

All-star nutrients

Vitamin K 662%

Vitamin A 220%

Vitamin C   66%

Folate   42%

Lutein & zeaxanthin ★

Serving size is 1 cup, cooked
Percent is Daily Value

And they're just bursting with vitamins A, C, and K. So for a major nutrition boost, join your Southern sisters in cooking greens, not just on New Year's but all year long, and enjoy a healthy addition to your meals.

Get an eyeful of cataract protection. Good news for your eyes — turnip greens and other leafy green veggies help protect them against cataracts. Leafy greens contain lutein and zeaxanthin. These unique nutrients are part of your eyes' defense system against cataract-causing damage from sunlight.

In the past, several large studies have suggested that shortages of lutein and zeaxanthin raise your risk of cataracts or cataract surgery. Here are the latest findings.

- An Australian study of more than 3,000 people age 40 and up suggests the more lutein and zeaxanthin in your diet, the less chance you'll suffer from cataracts.

- A 5-year Japanese study of 30,000 residents discovered that vitamin C might lower your odds of cataracts, too.

- Spanish research found that vitamin C, lutein, and zeaxanthin reduced the risk of cataracts in elderly nursing home residents.

Fortunately, turnip greens are rich in all three of these sight-saving nutrients. Similar "triple threat" foods include sweet peppers, Brussels sprouts, broccoli, and orange juice.

▪ ▪ ▪ ▪ ▪ Boost the benefits ▪ ▪ ▪ ▪ ▪

Don't boil turnip greens. Boiling leaches glucosinolates out of the turnip greens and into the cooking water. Because glucosinolates turn into cancer-fighting isothiocyanates, the cancer-busting power of turnip greens shrinks considerably without them. Instead, steam or sauté your turnip greens with oil and garlic, and then dress them with vinegar, pepper sauce, or lemon juice. And don't skip the oil. It helps you absorb more vitamin K, lutein, and zeaxanthin.

Benefit from other greens

Turnip greens aren't the only leafy greens that help fight cancer and other diseases. Just see how much nutrition you can get from these alternatives.

Greens (1 cup)	Lutein and zeaxanthin (mcg)	Vitamin A (IU)	Vitamin K (mcg)
kale	23720	17707	1062
collard	14619	15417	836
turnip	19541	10980	529
mustard	8347	8852	419
beet	2619	11022	697

Source: USDA National Nutrient Database for Standard Reference, Release 19

Ease hardening of the arteries. Turnip greens may not be the first heart-smart food you think of, but scientists suspect their lutein and vitamin K could help you avoid a heart attack. These nutrients may keep your heart from losing the one thing it can't live without — its fuel supply.

Your heart needs a constant supply of oxygen-rich blood to keep you alive and well. That's why you want to prevent clogs in the arteries leading to your heart. Those clogs get their start if harmful molecules called free radicals meet up with the "bad" LDL cholesterol in your bloodstream.

Together, these troublemakers coat the inside of your artery walls with a film called plaque. They also turn those same artery walls stiff and inflexible. These two effects may cause an artery-clogging blood clot, or plaque may just keep building up until it closes off the artery instead. Either blockage deprives your heart of vital fuel and could trigger a heart attack. But lutein and vitamin K can help prevent that.

Research shows that high lutein levels are linked to significantly less plaque build-up. Researchers also found a link between thicker artery walls — meaning more plaque — and low blood levels of lutein. So eating turnip greens and other high-lutein foods regularly may cut your heart attack risk.

What's more, experts suspect vitamin K may help prevent hardening of the arteries. Your body already has a special protein that may help keep your arteries from hardening, but that protein must have vitamin K to do its work. Ongoing research at the Jean Mayer USDA Human Nutrition Research Center on Aging will soon find out whether vitamin K affects arteries this way, so stay tuned.

Just remember, if you're taking warfarin or another blood-thinning medication, talk to your doctor before eating turnip greens and other foods rich in vitamin K.

Go "green" to stop cancer before it starts. A helping of turnip greens may not look like broccoli, but the turnip and its greens come from the same family of cancer fighters as broccoli and cabbage. And like broccoli, turnip greens contain glucosinolates, which break down into cancer-fighting isothiocyanates.

Isothiocyanates help keep normal cells from turning into cancer. Cancer-causing compounds in the foods you eat can damage the DNA in your cells — setting off a chain reaction that may change a normal cell into a cancer cell. But isothiocyanates defend your cells against DNA damage so cancerous changes can't get started. A Texas study found that people who ate the most isothiocyanates had nearly 30 percent less risk of bladder cancer.

But your cancer protection doesn't stop at isothiocyanates. Lutein and zeaxanthin lend a hand as well. Several studies have suggested lutein and zeaxanthin may cut your odds of lung cancer. For example, South Pacific islanders who ate lots of leafy greens had a lower rate of lung cancer than those who didn't. So take your cue from the healthy islanders, and eat delicious leafy greens like turnip greens, kale, and collard greens often.

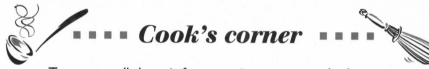

Cook's corner

To remove all the grit from turnip greens, put the leaves in cold water, stir, and let the water settle. Drain the gritty water and repeat. When you stop seeing grit in the water, the leaves are clean enough. Remove the stems before cooking.

Avoid cooking greens in aluminum pans or you'll spoil the flavor.

Keep turnip greens in a plastic bag in the fridge for up to five days.

Zucchini

Enjoy a lean green wellness machine

Both Thomas Jefferson and George Washington are said to have grown zucchini at their estates — not bad credentials for a humble green summer squash from Italy. But consider what it has to offer.

The zucchini is low calorie, fat free, and cholesterol free. Yet, it delivers manganese, vitamins A and C, and two blood pressure regulators — magnesium and potassium. Zucchini even gives you extra problem-solver

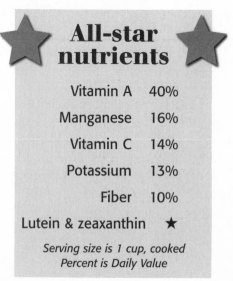

All-star nutrients

Vitamin A	40%
Manganese	16%
Vitamin C	14%
Potassium	13%
Fiber	10%
Lutein & zeaxanthin	★

Serving size is 1 cup, cooked
Percent is Daily Value

nutrients to fight against specific health problems. You'll learn more about those later in this chapter.

As if that weren't enough, zucchini is well suited to home gardens and delicious both raw and cooked. If you aren't already enjoying this versatile veggie, give it a try.

■ ■ ■ ■ ■ Boost the benefits ■ ■ ■ ■ ■

Don't peel your zucchini unless the skin is uncomfortably tough. All the zucchini's beta carotene is in the peel. Simply scrub the squash clean and cut off the ends. You can sauté slices in oil and garlic and add to pasta, or use as a side dish. Add raw slices to salads and sandwiches. They're good with dips, too.

Put the brakes on macular degeneration. Up to one quarter of people over age 65 show signs of age-related macular degeneration (AMD) — an eye disease that can cripple your eyesight or even cause blindness. Fortunately, summer squashes like zucchini contain a "magic formula" of nutrients that may help prevent AMD.

One of the key villains behind AMD is the blue, ultraviolet light that's part of sunlight. The phytochemicals lutein and zeaxanthin team up to shield your eyes against this light as well as the tissue damage it causes. A recent study of more than 4,000 people found that those who ate the most lutein and zeaxanthin had the least risk of macular degeneration. Because years of sunlight damage can lead to AMD, it's never too soon to begin protecting your eyes by getting more lutein and zeaxanthin in your diet.

Zucchini and other summer squash are a great place to start, but you should also include sources like corn, kale, winter squash, turnip greens, orange bell peppers, and spinach. For best results, eat these foods with a little healthy fat like olive oil. The fat helps your body absorb even more of these "magic" ingredients.

Discover the no-starve way to weight loss. You want to lose weight, but you think dieting would mean going hungry and giving up all your favorite Italian foods. Don't worry. You can eat until you're full, enjoy Italian treats, and still lose weight. Zucchini can help because it's high in both fiber and water.

Why is that important? Foods that are rich in water, fiber, or both usually have fewer calories per gram of weight. Research suggests that people eat the same amount of food, no matter what the calorie count. So a low-calorie meal high in fiber and water would satisfy you just as much as the high-calorie version. For example, if you replaced some of the high-fat cheese in a pasta dish with slices of zucchini, you'd still eat the same amount of food, but you'd feel full on fewer calories.

If you can't quite believe that, consider this. Fiber absorbs water, swells, and slows the movement of food through your upper digestive tract. When that happens, nerve receptors in your stomach send word to your brain that the stomach is full and you no longer need to eat. That makes you feel full even if you haven't eaten as many calories as you normally would. Adding fiber also makes protein and fat less digestible so you absorb fewer of those calories as well.

Water not only helps fiber do its job but may even pitch in extra help. Studies have shown that people who eat foods with high water content — like salads and soups — eat fewer calories from the meal that follows. So try replacing some of the calories and fat in your meals with high water, high-fiber foods like zucchini. You'll be more satisfied after meals, and the pounds will slip off more easily.

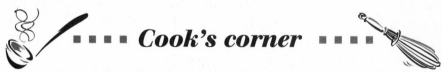

▪ ▪ ▪ ▪ *Cook's corner* ▪ ▪ ▪ ▪

The tastiest zucchinis are close to the length of a dollar bill, give or take a couple of inches.

Store regular-size zucchini in a plastic bag in your refrigerator crisper drawer for up to four days. The smaller "baby zucchini" may last only two days, so plan accordingly.

Try a plant-based diet for super health

Find the right vegetarian diet, and you may cut your risk of cavities, hemorrhoids, gallstones, diabetes, heart disease, cancer, and even obesity. Consider these options.

- **Flexitarian or semi-vegetarian.** Meals are at least 80 percent vegetarian. Occasionally eats meat, fish, poultry, eggs, milk, and cheese, but meals are mostly fruits, veggies, grains, and nuts.

- **Vegan.** Eats produce, nuts, and grains but no meat, fowl, fish, eggs, or dairy foods.

- **Ovo-vegetarian.** Similar to vegan but also includes eggs.

- **Lacto-vegetarian or Lacto-ovo-vegetarian.** Similar to vegan but dairy products and eggs are allowed.

- **Pescovegetarian.** Similar to vegan but includes seafood.

Meats, fish, and dairy products are the main source of some nutrients, so excluding these foods may cause dangerous deficiencies unless you plan carefully.

Vitamin B12 deficiency can cause nerve damage that may not be reversible. If you don't eat meat, find a cereal or plant food fortified with B12, or take a B12 supplement. Eat fortified cereals to help prevent such nutrient deficiencies as vitamin D, too. Meanwhile, get extra calcium from kale, broccoli, and fortified versions of rice milk or almond milk. Add zinc from foods like sunflower seeds, lima beans, whole grains, and brewer's yeast. And, unless you already take an iron supplement or multivitamin, eat iron-fortified foods and dried beans and peas.

But don't forget protein. It's more difficult to get enough protein from plants than meat, but you can combine foods to meet your daily requirement. Choose either grains or seeds, and then pair them up with beans, peas, or lentils. Try delicious red beans and rice to start.

Fruit: sweet treats yield big rewards

Avocados

■ ■ ■ ■ ■ ■ ■ ■ ■ ■ ■ ■ ■ ■

'Alligator pears' take bite out of poor health

Their bumpy texture and pear-like shape have given avocados the nickname "alligator pears" — and these tasty fruits are certainly worth snapping your jaws into. Packed with beneficial nutrients to fight a variety of conditions, avocados guard your health and please your taste buds.

Most avocados come from Mexico, but California and Florida also produce them. Hass avocados, the most common type, grow in Mexico and California and feature pebbly, purple-black skin and soft, buttery, green flesh. The larger Florida avocados have smooth green skin and half the fat of Hass avocados. They also do not have the same delicious flavor.

Avocados, whose name comes from the Aztec word for "testicle," have a long history. In fact, archaeologists in Peru discovered avocado pits in the tombs of Incan mummies dating back to 750 B.C.

You don't have to be an archaeologist to discover the many health benefits of avocados. Just keep reading to find out what avocados can do for you.

Shield yourself from heart problems. Just as their bumpy skin shields their yummy insides, avocados protect your heart. Thanks to a barrage of heart-healthy nutrients, your heart will fall in love with avocados.

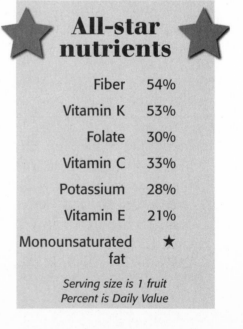

All-star nutrients

Fiber	54%
Vitamin K	53%
Folate	30%
Vitamin C	33%
Potassium	28%
Vitamin E	21%
Monounsaturated fat	★

Serving size is 1 fruit
Percent is Daily Value

■ ■ ■ ■ ■ Boost the benefits ■ ■ ■ ■ ■

When you think of avocado, you may think of guacamole. But there are healthier ways to enjoy this fabulous fruit. Instead of buttering your toast or slathering your sandwich with mayonnaise, spread on some mashed avocado. You'll get great taste without the saturated fat.

Add some diced avocado to your salads, and gain an extra edge. The healthy fat in avocados helps your body absorb nutrients like vitamins A, D, E, and K from the salad's other fruits and veggies. You can also make a healthy salad dressing by mixing avocado and balsamic vinegar.

- *Potassium.* This mineral plays an important role in regulating your blood pressure. It also helps lower your risk for stroke — probably because high blood pressure ranks as stroke's No. 1 risk factor. Good news — an avocado has more than twice as much potassium as a banana.

- *Fiber.* Like potassium, fiber also lowers your risk for stroke. Soluble fiber can also help lower cholesterol. Luckily, avocados contain both soluble and insoluble fiber.

- *Folate.* This B vitamin counteracts a substance called homocysteine that increases your risk of heart disease.

- *Monounsaturated fat.* Feel free to enjoy some guacamole at your next Super Bowl party. Shying away from avocados because of their high fat content is a mistake. These high-fat, "Super Bowl" fruits actually protect your good cholesterol and fight the bad, artery-clogging kind. That's because avocados contain mostly healthy monounsaturated fat. When you substitute monounsaturated fat for saturated fat, you can lower bad LDL cholesterol levels and boost your level of good HDL cholesterol.

■ *Vitamins C and E.* These antioxidant vitamins help prevent LDL cholesterol from becoming oxidized and, hence, more dangerous. Vitamin C may also help control blood pressure.

No wonder a recent study included avocados among the important fruits and vegetables that can reduce blood pressure and protect against both heart attack and stroke.

Avoid allergies

Allergic to latex? You may also react to avocado, which is related to the rubber plant.

Deal better with your diabetes. If you have diabetes, you should try to eat more avocados. In fact, the American Diabetes Association (ADA) recommends just that. Avocados give you a generous dose of monounsaturated fat, which makes a healthy substitute for saturated fat or even carbohydrates. Because they contain little or no carbohydrate, avocados do not even have a glycemic index value. That means they have almost no effect on your blood sugar. The ADA has found that a diet high in monounsaturated fat can improve glucose tolerance and may reduce insulin resistance, which can help you better control your disease.

In addition to their many heart benefits, avocados also help with weight control, another common concern for people with diabetes. Because monounsaturated fat fills you up and keeps you satisfied longer, you are less likely to overeat.

Avoid osteoporosis with stronger bones. Avocados are a surprisingly good source of vitamin K, a vitamin more commonly found in green, leafy vegetables. This vitamin helps protect your bones from osteoporosis. Studies link low vitamin K intake to lower bone mass density and higher risk of fractures. As a bonus, the potassium, magnesium, and vitamin C found in avocados may also help build bone mass and prevent bone loss and fractures.

Protect your prostate from cancer. With a name that means "testicle," it's no surprise avocados have a positive effect on men's health. A UCLA lab study found that avocado extract added to two types of prostate cancer cells inhibited cell growth by up to 60 percent. Avocados have several nutrients that can explain these results. Vitamin C and vitamin E help mop up free radicals that cause cell damage, and lutein, a carotenoid found in avocados that acts as an antioxidant, has been linked to a reduced risk of prostate cancer. Other possible contributors include the phytochemicals glutathione and beta-sitosterol.

Researchers at Ohio State University also found that avocado phytochemicals may help fight oral cancer. They believe they may eventually be linked to other cancers as well.

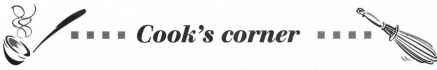

■ ■ ■ ■ *Cook's corner* ■ ■ ■ ■

■ When choosing an avocado, test for firmness, and avoid fruits with shriveled or puckered skin. To speed up the ripening process, you can put an avocado in a paper bag. Its natural ethylene gas does the trick.

■ Avocados brown quickly after being cut, but drizzling lemon or lime juice on them helps prevent that. It also adds some flavor.

■ You can serve avocados several ways. Serve slices with cooked food, dice and mix into salads, mash to make toppings or dips, or even purée in cold soups or desserts. Just don't cook avocados or they become bitter.

Bananas

For better health, just peel and heal

Why monkey around with pills? Just peel a banana and reap the many health benefits of this tropical fruit. Bananas rank as the leading fresh fruit sold in the United States. These curved fruits grow in bunches, or hands, on banana trees — which are technically tree-like herbs belonging to the grass family. A banana plant can grow up to 40 feet tall.

India, Brazil, the Philippines, Ecuador, and Indonesia produce most of the world's bananas, but the United States also grows them. The most popular variety, the Cavendish, sports a yellow peel and soft, white, sweet, fragrant flesh. Packed with potassium, manganese, vitamin C, vitamin B6, and fiber, bananas provide more than just good taste.

Indian legend says a banana — not an apple — was the fruit offered to Adam in the Garden of Eden, so bananas are called the "fruit of paradise" in India. Whatever you call them, bananas make a handy, portable, healthy snack. Just be careful not to slip on the peel!

Sweet treat battles high blood pressure. If you don't take precautions, your blood pressure can climb higher than a banana tree. Luckily, the fruit of that tree can help. In fact, an Indian study found that eating two bananas a day can lower blood pressure by 10 percent. That's because bananas provide plenty of potassium and barely any sodium. This winning combination keeps your blood pressure under control.

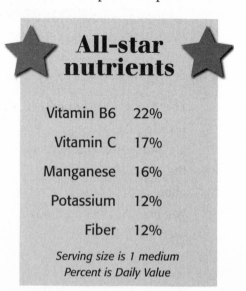

All-star nutrients

Vitamin B6	22%
Vitamin C	17%
Manganese	16%
Potassium	12%
Fiber	12%

Serving size is 1 medium
Percent is Daily Value

It also gives bananas the Food and Drug Administration (FDA) seal of approval. The FDA allows banana producers to make the following health claim: "Diets containing foods that are a good source of potassium and that are low in sodium may reduce the risk of high blood pressure and stroke."

Studies show a potassium-rich diet can reduce the risk of stroke by 22 to 40 percent. Recent guidelines of the Institute of Medicine recommend getting at least 4.7 grams (4,700 mg) of potassium a day. The Dietary Approaches to Stop Hypertension (DASH) diet also recommends 4,700 mg of potassium — and includes plenty of fruits and vegetables, like bananas. A medium-sized banana gives you about 420 mg of potassium.

While potassium gets much of the credit, other nutrients in bananas contribute as well. A recent Tulane analysis of 25 studies found that boosting your fiber intake can significantly lower your blood pressure. People who benefited ate between 7 and 19 grams of fiber a day for at least eight weeks. One medium banana gives you 3 grams of fiber. Vitamin C may also help with high blood pressure by keeping your arteries flexible.

■ ■ ■ ■ ■ Boost the benefits ■ ■ ■ ■ ■

Boost your energy by knowing what to eat. Start your day by topping your breakfast cereal with sliced bananas. This fruity, high fiber breakfast is a great way to keep your energy up throughout a busy morning.

As you start to drag during the afternoon, a banana is the perfect snack to help keep your brain sharp. After all, a banana provides all the nutrients of an energy bar — without the extra calories or extra cost. And munching on a banana about an hour before you exercise will give you the energy you need to make it through your workout.

Relieve the discomfort of diarrhea. You're spending a lot of time on the throne, but you sure don't feel like a king or queen. Get royal relief from diarrhea and other gastrointestinal problems with bananas.

Bananas serve as the perfect food after a bout of diarrhea or vomiting. Once you can eat solid food again, soft, bland foods like bananas give you the nutrients you need without upsetting your stomach.

Even if you have a more serious condition, like colitis, bananas can be an important part of a safe, bland diet. The potassium in bananas also helps protect your intestine. More protection may come from substances called fructo-oligosaccharides (FOS). Also known as prebiotics, these molecules stimulate the growth of probiotics, good bacteria that ward off harmful bacteria.

One study found that green bananas — which are different from unripe bananas — might help treat children with persistent diarrhea. Bananas can also help thicken your stool, which helps prevent fecal incontinence, or loss of bowel control.

Avoid osteoporosis with bone-bolstering mineral. Watching someone slip on a banana peel in an old movie may be funny, but the risk of falling associated with osteoporosis is no laughing matter. To protect yourself from osteoporosis, or brittle bone disease, watch out for the peel, and eat the rest of the banana.

A University of California San Francisco study found that potassium helps prevent calcium loss caused by a high-salt diet. This important mineral may also counteract the negative effects of a high-protein diet. Vitamin C and manganese also play key roles in bone health.

Knock out painful kidney stones. Avoid the pain of kidney stones with an extra helping of bananas. Foods rich in potassium may reduce your risk of developing this condition. In fact, studies show that a high intake of potassium, from a diet rich in fruits and vegetables, can slash your risk of stones by 30 to 50 percent.

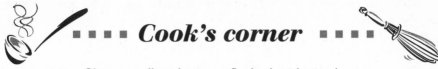

Cook's corner

- Choose yellow bananas flecked with tiny brown specks, which are a sign of ripeness. Avoid mushy or damaged fruits or those with green tips.

- If you need to speed up the ripening process, you can put bananas in a paper bag or wrap them in newspaper. You should not refrigerate bananas, but you can freeze them for later use.

- Bananas turn brown when exposed to air. To prevent this, brush the banana with lemon or lime juice, or dip it in acidulated water — cold water with a splash of vinegar or citrus juice.

Blueberries

'Berry' good benefits come in small packages

Blueberries appeared on North America long before American settlers, who took their cue from the Indians and used these sweet, juicy berries as both food and medicine.

You can find over 50 species of blueberries, both cultivated and wild, with shades varying from light blue to dark purple. Blueberries are cultivated mainly in Canada and the United States. These cultivated berries are larger and sweeter than wild blueberries, which are more tart. But all of these tiny fruits pack plenty of powerful nutrients, including vitamin C, vitamin K, and manganese, and antioxidants like polyphenols and anthocyanins.

In the berry world, blueberries rank second, behind only strawberries, in terms of popularity. But these little dynamos take a back seat to no one. After all, blueberries used to be called star berries. Although that nickname came from the star-shaped calyx on top of each fruit, it could just as easily refer to the blueberry's nutritional star power when it comes to your health.

Give your brain a powerful boost. Remember to eat your blueberries. They can help you remember everything else. That's because blueberries are chock-full of polyphenols that benefit your brain.

In a recent study, a flavonol called epicatechin found in blueberries — as well as chocolate and other fruits and vegetables — improved memory in mice. Other studies have shown that blueberries, thanks to their antioxidant polyphenols, can reverse normal age-related declines in brain signaling and improve thinking and motor skills. In other words, simply eating blueberries can help you keep your brain sharp as you get older.

Blueberries may also protect you from stroke and help limit the damage and speed up recovery if you suffer one. They may even help ward off Alzheimer's disease. You can also slash your risk of Alzheimer's with strawberries, another antioxidant-rich berry that has shown promise in studies. While most of these studies involved animals, scientists are working on proving the blueberry's benefit to people as well. If these tiny fruits can help aging rats navigate through a maze, they may help you balance your checkbook or remember where you left your car keys.

Berries burst with cancer protection. The same pigments that give blueberries their bright blue color could also protect you against cancer, particularly of the

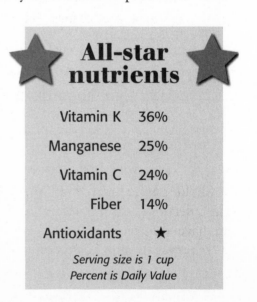

All-star nutrients

Vitamin K	36%
Manganese	25%
Vitamin C	24%
Fiber	14%
Antioxidants	★

Serving size is 1 cup
Percent is Daily Value

colon. Researchers at the University of Georgia found that anthocyanins in blueberries significantly inhibited the growth of two types of colon cancer cells. Anthocyanins may also trigger apoptosis — the death of cancer cells. Other substances in blueberries, including flavonols and tannins, also helped thwart colon cancer cells to a lesser degree.

Another antioxidant substance in blueberries called pterostilbene has also shown promising results against colon cancer in lab studies of rats. It may work by reducing lipids, or fats, in the blood. Previous studies have shown that pterostilbene can lower cholesterol. Other researchers have found that blueberry extracts helped fight esophageal cancer in rodents and oral and prostate cancer in test tube studies.

Vitamin C, an antioxidant vitamin, and fiber — both found in blueberries — have also been linked to cancer prevention. Eating more blueberries, as well as other fruits and vegetables, may help guard against this dreaded disease. Aim for two cups of blueberries a week for optimum protection.

■ ■ ■ ■ ■ Boost the benefits ■ ■ ■ ■ ■

Whether you eat them fresh or dried, blueberries make the perfect snack on their own. But you can find several other ways to fit more of these fabulous fruits into your diet.

For instance, sprinkle some blueberries onto your breakfast cereal, or add them to your salads, yogurt, or ice cream. Blend blueberries into refreshing smoothies, or purée them to make tasty jams or jellies. You can also use them in pancakes, muffins, pies, breads, syrup, and sauces.

Shake off bacteria that cause UTIs. When it comes to urinary tract infections, cranberries get most of the publicity. But blueberries can have the same protective effect, thanks to proanthocyanidins. These powerful antioxidant compounds prevent bacteria from sticking to the cells that line your urinary tract. Blueberries may also increase the acidity of your urine, which helps destroy harmful bacteria.

Easy way to enhance your eyesight. Blueberries may be a treat for your taste buds, but they're also a sight for sore eyes. The bilberry, a European version of the blueberry, has been linked to improved eyesight in several European studies. Its power comes from the anthocyanins that give the bilberry its dark blue color. Because blueberries also pack plenty of anthocyanins, they should also safeguard your vision. In fact, a Japanese study found that blueberries can help ease eye fatigue. Make brightly colored foods like blueberries a part of your diet, and you'll see plenty of benefits.

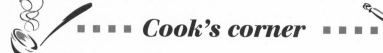

■ ■ ■ ■ *Cook's corner* ■ ■ ■ ■

Choose firm, large, plump blueberries. They should have a purple-blue to blue-black color with a silver frost. Stay away from green, dull, or mushy berries.

If they come in a container, tilt the container to check if the berries move freely. If they stick together, they could be moldy. Also make sure the container is dry and unstained.

Refrigerate blueberries, unwashed, for up to six days. Rinse blueberries very briefly in cold water before using them. You can also freeze blueberries in their cardboard container for later use.

Good nutrition from a can

Nothing beats the taste of fresh, seasonal produce. But you don't need to buy fresh fruits and vegetables to reap their benefits. Canned and frozen varieties also boost your health. In fact, they are just as nutritious as fresh produce. Sometimes, they're even better. Canned tomatoes, for instance, have much more lycopene than fresh tomatoes. All food loses some vitamins during processing, but so does fresh produce that sits in the grocery store or your refrigerator too long. Food frozen or canned at its peak could have more nutrients than fresh produce. Buying these items is an easy, cheap way to enjoy your favorite produce out of season.

Canned fruits come with extra calories if they come packed in sugary syrup. Choose those packed in their own juices instead. Read labels, and skip canned foods with too much salt or sugar added. Rinse canned vegetables to get rid of extra salt. Avoid frozen packages with ice crystals or signs of refreezing, and stay away from dusty, dented, or bulging cans. Buy frozen foods right before checking out and take them straight home.

Once there, keep everything from strawberries to onions fresh days or weeks longer with these simple tips. Store fresh strawberries, unwashed, in a colander in your refrigerator. Wrap onions in aluminum foil to keep them from sprouting. Put a dry sponge in the crisper to absorb moisture. Forget freezer burn when you follow these tips for frost-free frozen food. Pack fruits like strawberries in simple syrup to reduce the formation of ice crystals. Blanching vegetables will do the same thing. Put items in labeled, dated, plastic freezer bags, and squeeze all the air out. For even more protection, put that bag in a second freezer bag before storing.

Cherries

■ ■ ■ ■ ■ ■ ■ ■ ■ ■ ■ ■

Sweet or sour, tiny fruit packs power

Life may not always be a bowl of cherries — but an occasional bowl of cherries could make your life healthier.

Cherries come in sweet and tart varieties. Both kinds provide vitamin C, fiber, and potassium. They are also loaded with antioxidants. Tart, or sour, cherries also give you lots of vitamin A as well as copper and manganese.

The juicy Bing cherry is the most popular sweet cherry, while common tart varieties include Montmorency, Morello, and Balaton. These dark red tart fruits are usually cooked rather than eaten raw.

In the United States, most cherry trees grow in Michigan, but cherries also come from Washington, Oregon, Idaho, New York, Pennsylvania, Wisconsin, and Utah. One cherry tree can yield more than 100 pounds of fruit each season.

The Food and Drug Administration (FDA) has clamped down on cherry producers who make health claims, but that doesn't mean cherries aren't chock full of benefits. Check out what these sweet and sour treats can do for you.

Knock out the pain of gout. Cherries have long been a popular folk remedy for gout. New research from the U.S. Department of Agriculture supports the use of cherries to treat this painful condition.

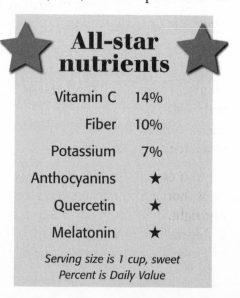

All-star nutrients

Vitamin C	14%
Fiber	10%
Potassium	7%
Anthocyanins	★
Quercetin	★
Melatonin	★

Serving size is 1 cup, sweet
Percent is Daily Value

In a recent study, 10 women each ate 45 fresh, pitted Bing cherries. Five hours later, their blood levels of urate — a substance your body converts to uric acid, which contributes to gout — were significantly lower. At the same time, more urate showed up in their urine, meaning they had flushed it from their body. Their blood levels of C-reactive protein and nitric oxide, two common markers of inflammation, also decreased slightly.

Compounds in cherries may block inflammatory pathways, making cherries a good weapon against not only gout but other inflammatory conditions as well.

Earlier laboratory studies found that the anthocyanins in cherries — the pigments that give cherries their red color — helped suppress inflammation. In fact, cherries were 10 times more effective than aspirin in treating arthritis pain and inflammation. They also come without the harmful side effects of nonsteroidal anti-inflammatory drugs (NSAIDS).

Folk remedies include eating six to eight fresh cherries a day to relieve the symptoms of gout. If you feel a bout of gout coming on, try eating 20 to 30 cherries right away. Cherries may even help sore muscles recover after a workout.

If you can't get fresh cherries, dried cherries and cherry juice should also do the trick.

Enjoy a sweet path to sounder sleep. Tart cherries may provide sweet dreams. Researchers recently discovered that cherries contain melatonin, a natural hormone essential to your body's sleep cycle.

As one of the few food sources of melatonin, cherries could act as an antidote to insomnia. Experts say eating a handful of tart cherries before bed may boost melatonin levels and promote a more restful sleep. Melatonin, an antioxidant, may also help you overcome jet lag or adjust to a late-shift work schedule.

You can also boost your energy by knowing how to nap. A nap can be as short as five minutes or as long as two hours. Usually, 20 minutes is just right. The best time to nap is early in the afternoon. Choose a dark, comfortable room for your nap, but make sure to wake up at least three hours before bedtime so you don't interfere with your nighttime sleep.

■ ■ ■ ■ ■ **Boost the benefits** ■ ■ ■ ■ ■

Sure, cherries make tasty pies, jams, and other sweet goodies. But you can find better ways to fit these healthy fruits into your diet.

Dried cherries, which make a great snack, are especially versatile. Add dried cherries to trail mix, cereal, oatmeal, yogurt, or pancakes. You can also use them in muffins, couscous, rice pilaf, risotto, pasta, and tossed or fruit salads. When working out, swap your usual energy bar for half a cup of dried cherries instead.

For a refreshing beverage, mix cherry juice concentrate with water or seltzer water. Or blend frozen cherries with cherry juice concentrate and yogurt for a cool treat.

Nutrients may provide an answer to cancer. Cherries certainly don't look intimidating. But these little, round, red fruits may make cancer cells quake in their boots. That's because cherries contain several substances to fight cancer.

Anthocyanins and cyanidin, two flavonoids found in cherries, have shown promise against colon cancer in animal studies and laboratory studies of human cancer cells. These flavonoids inhibit tumor development and help stop colon cancer cell growth.

Perillyl alcohol, a phytonutrient found in cherries, thwarts the development and progression of cancer. Studies have found it helps treat or prevent breast, prostate, lung, liver, and skin cancers.

Cherries also contain known cancer fighters like ellagic acid and quercetin. And they provide fiber and vitamin C — key ingredients in any healthy, anti-cancer diet.

Give your heart tip-top protection. Because the anthocyanins in cherries fight inflammation, they may also protect you from heart disease. One sign of inflammation is a substance called C-reactive protein (CRP) — which may be a more important indicator of heart disease risk than high LDL cholesterol.

In a recent study, 18 healthy men and women ate about 45 fresh, pitted Bing cherries a day for 28 days. After 28 days, their blood levels of CRP plummeted by 25 percent. Less CRP in the blood means less inflammation and a lower risk of heart disease. They also had lower levels of nitric oxide, another marker of inflammation.

Other nutrients in cherries, such as potassium, which regulates blood pressure; vitamin C; and fiber also do wonders for your heart's health.

Delicious way to head off diabetes. Cherries just might hold the key to beating obesity and diabetes. In a recent lab study, researchers at Michigan State University put some mice on a high-fat diet and others on a low-fat diet. The high-fat mice quickly gained weight, developed fatty livers, and became glucose intolerant. Researchers then began feeding them anthocyanins, compounds found in cherries, in addition to their fatty food. After eight weeks, these obese, glucose-intolerant mice had lost weight, lowered their cholesterol, raised their insulin levels, were more glucose-sensitive, and once again had healthy livers. The researchers used Cornelian cherries but say the more popular tart cherries are similar.

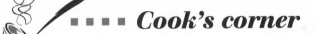

▪ ▪ ▪ ▪ *Cook's corner* ▪ ▪ ▪ ▪

- Buy organic cherries whenever possible. You will pay more, but the extra cost may be worth it. That's because cherries are among the fruits and vegetables most likely to have high levels of pesticide residues on them.

- Choose brightly colored, plump, firm cherries. Stay away from small, pale, hard cherries as well as soft ones with brownish spots or bruised or shriveled skin.

- You can refrigerate cherries for up to one week or freeze them for up to one year. They tend to absorb odors, though, so keep them away from strong-smelling foods.

- Rinse cherries under cool water before using. To pit cherries, buy a simple cherry pitter or cut them in half. Be careful, though. They can stain your hands or clothes.

Cranberries

■ ■ ■ ■ ■ ■ ■ ■ ■ ■ ■ ■ ■ ■ ■ ■

Give thanks for berry's healing power

No Thanksgiving dinner would be complete without cranberry sauce — not even the first one. Native to North America, these tart red cousins of the blueberry were part of the original Thanksgiving feast. In fact, Indians not only ate cranberries, they used them as dyes and poultices for wounds. Later, American whalers and seamen brought cranberries — a good source of vitamin C — on their voyages to ward off scurvy.

Most cranberries come from Massachusetts, but Wisconsin, New Jersey, Washington, Oregon, and Canada also produce them. Cranberries grow on vines planted in sandy bogs. This allows growers to cover the plants with water to protect them from the cold.

But there's no need to get "bogged" down in further details. Just be thankful for all the wonderful ways cranberries protect your health.

Stop urinary tract infections. Drinking cranberry juice is an old folk remedy for urinary tract infections (UTIs). No wonder it has stood the test of time — it really works.

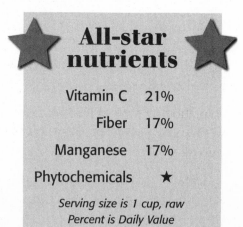

All-star nutrients

Vitamin C	21%
Fiber	17%
Manganese	17%
Phytochemicals	★

Serving size is 1 cup, raw
Percent is Daily Value

146

Several studies have found that cranberry juice can prevent and even treat UTIs. One study of nursing home residents found that drinking 4 to 6 ounces of cranberry juice each day for seven weeks prevented UTIs in two-thirds of the residents.

A Finnish study found that cranberry juice was much more effective than a probiotic drink in preventing UTIs. Even bacteria that have developed a resistance to antibiotics meet their match with cranberry juice.

Compounds called proanthocyanidins, or condensed tannins, give cranberries their power over UTIs. That's because they prevent bacteria from sticking to the walls of your urinary tract. Tannins may work by crushing tiny hairs on the bacteria's surface so they can't attach to the cells in the urinary tract.

You don't even have to get your cranberries in liquid form. A recent study reports that dried cranberries may also work.

To ward off UTIs, many health professionals recommend drinking two or three 8-ounce glasses of unsweetened cranberry juice a day. Or you can eat about a third of a cup of dried cranberries.

Counteract cancer with phytochemicals. Cranberries are loaded with phytochemicals that team up to fight cancer. The proanthocyanidins in cranberries — the compounds that make cranberries effective against urinary tract infections — also inhibit lung, colon, and leukemia cells in lab tests. They may even help improve existing cancer treatments. In a recent study, cranberry juice extract made platinum-based chemotherapy, the standard treatment for ovarian cancer, six times more effective.

Quercetin, a flavonoid abundant in cranberries, thwarts breast, colon, pancreatic, and leukemia cancer cells. Ursolic acid, found in the peel of cranberries, stops tumor growth of colon, prostate, lung, cervical, and leukemia cells.

Anthocyanins, the pigments that give cranberries their red color, also may give you an edge against cancer. They may fight inflammation, reducing your risk of developing certain cancers.

Researchers aren't sure exactly how each phytochemical fights cancer. Likely mechanisms include triggering apoptosis, or cancer cell death, stopping reproduction and colony formation, and limiting the cancer's ability to invade and spread. But one thing is sure — when you add it all up, cranberries pack one heck of a punch against cancer.

> ■ ■ ■ ■ ■ **Boost the benefits** ■ ■ ■ ■ ■
>
> While cranberries are usually too tart to eat raw, you can still find several ways to get them into your diet. They make great juice drinks, dried snacks, sauces, relishes, jams, and chutneys. You can also bake them into muffins or breads or sprinkle dried cranberries over your hot oatmeal or cold cereal.
>
> One way to counteract the tartness of cranberries is to blend them with other fruits, like oranges, apples, pears, or pineapples. Try baking your next apple pie with half cranberries and half apples.
>
> You can even take advantage of their tartness by using them in salads instead of vinegar. Just toss the greens with olive oil and add a handful of raw cranberries.

Safeguard your heart. The high polyphenol content of cranberries means plenty of good news for your heart.

Tests show that cranberry extracts, rich in flavonoids like quercetin, myrecetin, and anthocyanidins, inhibit the oxidation of LDL, or bad cholesterol. If LDL particles do not become oxidized, they can't do damage to your artery walls. As an added bonus, cranberry juice may also help boost your levels of HDL, or good cholesterol.

In one study of pigs, cranberry juice powder helped improve the ability of blood vessels to relax. Of course, you don't have to be a pig to reap the heart-healthy benefits of cranberries. Just "pig out" on these delicious fruits.

Overcome ulcers. The same mechanism that helps cranberries prevent urinary tract infections also helps them foil ulcers.

Just as cranberry juice prevents the *E. coli* bacteria from sticking to the walls of your urinary tract, this tasty beverage also works against *H. pylori,* the bacteria responsible for ulcers. If *H. pylori* can't stick to the mucus lining your stomach, it can't colonize there.

Even if you already have an *H. pylori* infection, cranberry juice may help. In a Chinese study, people who had *H. pylori* infections drank either two juice boxes of cranberry juice or a placebo beverage each day for 90 days. At the end of the study, those drinking the cranberry juice had significantly more negative test results for the infection.

Protect your teeth and gums. Smile if you like cranberries. Considering all they do for your mouth, it's hard to suppress a grin.

A Japanese study found that cranberries stop the oral streptococci strains of bacteria from sticking to the surface of your teeth. This slows the development of dental plaque and tooth decay. Researchers at the University of Rochester also found that cranberry juice effectively countered oral bacteria. They credited quercetin, as well as proanthocyanidins, for cranberry juice's success.

Just remember to drink unsweetened cranberry juice. Otherwise, the added sugar may do your teeth more harm than good.

▪ ▪ ▪ ▪ *Cook's corner* ▪ ▪ ▪ ▪

Cranberries used to be called bounceberries, because they bounce when ripe. Fortunately, you don't have to bounce cranberries to find good ones. Just look for brightly colored, firm, plump berries. Avoid pale, mushy, or wrinkled fruits.

You can store cranberries in the refrigerator for up to a month or freeze them for several months.

Cook cranberries in a small amount of water and keep the pot uncovered. Otherwise, steam will cause them to swell and explode like popcorn.

Figs

■ ■ ■ ■ ■ ■ ■

Embrace flower power for good health

Mithridates, king of the ancient Greek city of Pontus, considered figs an antidote for all ailments and even ordered his citizens to eat figs daily. There have certainly been worse laws. These sweet, chewy treats are loaded with fiber and polyphenols. They also provide potassium, manganese, vitamin B6, vitamin K, and calcium.

While considered a fruit, figs are actually inverted flowers. Their tiny seeds, which add a pleasant texture, are the true fruits of the fig tree. American figs come from California, while Turkey, Greece, Portugal, and Spain also rank among the top fig producers.

You may know figs from the Fig Newton cookie, one of the first commercially baked products in the United States. But they were a popular snack long before that. The Bible contains several references to this highly regarded food, which was also Cleopatra's favorite fruit. In fact, the asp that killed her was hidden in a basket of figs. Chances are, you won't find any poisonous snakes among your figs — but you will find a wealth of health benefits.

Conquer constipation naturally. Instead of relying on laxatives, try nature's cure for constipation — fiber. Fiber helps move things along in your intestines by bulking up and softening your stools.

Eat more figs, and you'll get more fiber. Just two medium figs give you nearly 3 grams of fiber,

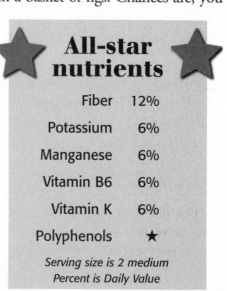

All-star nutrients

Fiber	12%
Potassium	6%
Manganese	6%
Vitamin B6	6%
Vitamin K	6%
Polyphenols	★

*Serving size is 2 medium
Percent is Daily Value*

or 12 percent of the recommended Daily Value. Dried figs pack even more fiber into a smaller package. One cup of dried figs provides 15 grams of fiber, or a whopping 58 percent of the Daily Value.

Figs may improve your digestive health in other ways, too. That's because adding more fiber to your diet may also help fight hemorrhoids, diverticular disease, irritable bowel syndrome (IBS), and colon cancer.

Just remember to add fiber to your diet gradually. Adding too much fiber too quickly may lead to gas and bloating. You also want to make sure to drink plenty of water when eating a high-fiber diet.

■ ■ ■ ■ ■ **Boost the benefits** ■ ■ ■ ■ ■

There's a lot more to figs than just the Fig Newton. You can add sliced figs to green salads for sweetness, texture, and added fiber. You can also use them as pizza toppings. They make good desserts, too. Just dip fresh figs in yogurt using the stem as a handle.

Sprinkle chopped, dried figs on squash before baking or on your cold cereal or oatmeal. Figs also go well with pasta or cooked grains, like barley, couscous, or brown rice. You can even puree figs to use as a substitute for oil in baked goods.

Keep your weight in check. Maybe you want to shed a few pounds. Or just keep off the weight you've already lost. Either way, that sweet tooth of yours makes weight control a hefty challenge.

Look no further than figs. These tasty treats can satisfy your craving for something sweet — without any fat. That combination makes figs an ideal snack for people trying to control their weight.

The fiber in figs also fills you up quickly and keeps you full for a while, so you're less likely to overeat. And, because your body can't digest fiber, it passes through your system without adding extra calories.

Ward off cancer. Adam and Eve covered themselves with fig leaves in the Garden of Eden. These days, you can find better ways to shield your body — but figs may still shield you from cancer.

A recent study at the University of Scranton found that figs — especially dried figs — were practically bursting with antioxidant polyphenols. These substances have been linked to both heart disease and cancer prevention. In an Israeli laboratory study, compounds isolated from fig resin strongly suppressed the spread of various cancer cells.

Experts also recommend boosting your fiber intake to guard against certain types of cancer. Eating more fiber-rich figs is an easy way to do that.

Give your heart a helping hand. Instead of gold medals, winners of ancient Olympic events received figs as awards. When it comes to your heart's health, a fig is still quite a prize. Here's what makes figs so special.

- *Polyphenols.* With more antioxidant polyphenols than red wine or tea, figs actively fight heart disease. These polyphenols help prevent LDL, or bad cholesterol, from becoming oxidized, a key step in the formation of plaque in the walls of your arteries.

- *Potassium.* This important mineral helps keep your blood pressure under control. It also helps lower your risk of stroke.

- *Calcium.* Like potassium, calcium helps regulate your blood pressure.

- *Fiber.* Figs contain both insoluble fiber and cholesterol-lowering soluble fiber.

▪ ▪ ▪ ▪ *Cook's corner* ▪ ▪ ▪ ▪

Choose plump, fairly soft figs that smell sweet. Their stems should be intact. Avoid dry, green, or bruised fruits. Always handle these delicate fruits carefully.

You can refrigerate figs, which are quite perishable, for a few days. Just make sure to wrap them well so they don't absorb odors. You can also freeze them for up to one year.

If you have overripe or damaged figs, don't despair. You can still stew them, cook them, or use them for baking.

Turn grocery shopping into a supermarket bonanza

Knowing which foods are healthy is important. But knowing how to save money on these foods is priceless. Find out how to trim your grocery bills by as much as $50 to $150 a month without cutting back on food. Just follow these helpful tips.

- **Make sure price is right.** Learn the prices of common items, so you know a good deal when you see it. Pay attention to the price per unit so you can more effectively compare prices.

- **Bend for bargains.** The most popular and expensive items are at eye level. Shop the bottom shelves for deals.

- **Time it right.** Shop on Tuesdays or Wednesdays, when supermarkets run most of their specials and stores are less crowded.

- **Go generic.** Generic or store brands are often just as good — and cheaper — than high-end products.

- **Scale back.** Ask the store to break up bunches of produce so you can buy a smaller amount. Don't pay for more than you will eat.

- **Walk past gimmicks.** Supermarkets display items at the ends of aisles to make you think they are a special deal. They're usually not.

- **Shop seasonally.** When markets have an abundance of certain foods, prices drop.

- **Get inside tips.** Chat with your grocers. You may find out about special deals from stocking clerks, butchers, and store managers.

- **Double-check at checkout.** Watch the register and check receipts. Mistakes can happen. A checker may scan an item twice or the sale price may not ring up.

Grapefruit

■■■■■■■■■■■■■■■■■■■

Large citrus fruit big on benefits

In a famous scene from the movie "The Public Enemy," James Cagney shoves a grapefruit in Mae Clarke's face. But this delicious citrus fruit deserves more than a mere cameo. With its vast supply of vitamin C, plus vitamin A, potassium, and fiber, the grapefruit merits a leading role in your diet.

A cross between a pomelo and an orange, grapefruit is one of the largest citrus fruits. It comes in white, pink, and red varieties and has a refreshingly tart taste. Like all citrus fruits, it also features segmented flesh.

Grapefruit grow in clusters, like grapes, which probably explains how the fruit got its name. Most grapefruit grow in Florida, Texas, and California, but they also come from South America, Mexico, Israel, and Mediterranean countries.

No matter where you get your grapefruit, make sure to treat it — and your breakfast companion — with more respect than Cagney did. In return, this amazing fruit can help you lower your cholesterol, lose weight, and even avoid cancer.

Chop down high cholesterol. A grapefruit a day keeps high cholesterol away. That's what Israeli researchers discovered in a recent study.

The 30-day study involved 57 people with high cholesterol, randomly divided into three groups. In one group, participants ate one red grapefruit each

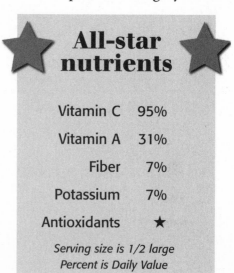

All-star nutrients

Vitamin C	95%
Vitamin A	31%
Fiber	7%
Potassium	7%
Antioxidants	★

Serving size is 1/2 large
Percent is Daily Value

day, while the people in another group ate a white grapefruit of equal size. The third group served as the control group and did not eat any grapefruit.

■ ■ ■ ■ ■ **Boost the benefits** ■ ■ ■ ■ ■

Breakfast may be the most important meal of the day, but it's not the only time to enjoy grapefruit. Get more from this great fruit by using it in different ways.

Serve grapefruit halves as a first course for dinner or use grapefruit in fruit or vegetable salads, vinaigrettes, and sorbets. Grilled grapefruit goes well with chicken, duck, pork, and shrimp dishes. Substitute grapefruit for oranges or pineapples in many recipes. You can even lightly sprinkle half a grapefruit with sugar and broil it for dessert.

Both grapefruit groups showed tremendous improvement in their cholesterol levels, but those eating red grapefruit fared the best. They slashed total cholesterol by 15.5 percent, LDL cholesterol by 20.3 percent, and triglycerides by 17.2 percent. The white grapefruit group lowered total cholesterol by 7.6 percent, LDL cholesterol by 10.7 percent, and triglycerides by 5.6 percent.

The many antioxidants in grapefruit — including vitamins C and A — probably deserve the credit for their cholesterol-lowering effect. The fiber and potassium in grapefruit also serve your heart well.

You don't need to know exactly why grapefruit works. Just remember this simple bit of math. Add a daily grapefruit to your diet, and you'll subtract cholesterol.

Knock out kidney stones. Few things are more painful than kidney stones. Luckily, preventing them can be painless. Just drink more grapefruit juice.

An Italian study found that grapefruit juice not only boosted urinary flow, it also significantly increased the levels of citrate, calcium, and magnesium in the urine. That means grapefruit juice could be a safer, cheaper alternative to drugs like potassium citrate for the management of kidney stones. For best results, look for a juice with reduced sugar.

German researchers also found that grapefruit juice reduced the risk of kidney stone formation. Apple juice and orange juice also lessened the risk.

Citrus fruit blocks certain cancers. When it comes to grapefruit and cancer, there's good news and bad news. An Italian analysis of several nutrition studies found that citrus fruit, like grapefruit, helps protect you from oral cancer. Just eating one citrus fruit a day can lower your risk of mouth cancer by 62 percent. While other fruits and vegetables also help, citrus fruits provided the most protection.

Grapefruit may also fight prostate cancer, according to a recent laboratory study. Pectin, a type of complex carbohydrate found in citrus fruits, helps correct miscommunication between prostate cells that can lead to cancer. It may also help battle other cancers. For best results, eat the whole fruit rather than just the juice. The meat of the fruit and the membrane that separates the segments contain the highest concentration of pectin.

Alas, grapefruit may also increase your risk of breast cancer because it raises your estrogen levels. A recent study found that eating one-quarter of a grapefruit or more each day boosts the risk of breast cancer by 30 percent in postmenopausal women.

Sidestep dangerous drug interactions

Sometimes a healthy food can be dangerous. That's what happens when you mix grapefruit or grapefruit juice with certain prescription drugs, including calcium channel blockers for high blood pressure, cholesterol-lowering statins, and drugs for anxiety, insomnia, or depression.

Chemicals in grapefruit called furanocoumarins are responsible for the interaction, which results in higher levels of the drug in your bloodstream — and potentially dangerous side effects. Ask your doctor if your medication is safe to take with grapefruit or grapefruit juice.

Easy way to control your weight. Fad grapefruit diets often promise unbelievable — and impossible — results. But a recent study at the Scripps Clinic in San Diego found that grapefruit really does help you lose weight.

People who ate half a grapefruit three times a day, before each meal, lost an average of 3.6 pounds over the 12-week study. Some lost as much as 10 pounds. They also showed slight improvements in their insulin levels, meaning grapefruit may also reduce your risk of diabetes. Drinking an 8-ounce glass of grapefruit juice three times a day also led to modest weight loss, an average of 3.3 pounds.

Grapefruit may help control your weight in a number of ways. Lowering your insulin level makes you feel less hungry. Plus, naringin, a compound in grapefruit, slows enzymes in the small intestine that help metabolize some fats and carbohydrates. The high water and fiber content of grapefruit may also help fill you up, so you're less likely to overeat.

▪ ▪ ▪ ▪ *Cook's corner* ▪ ▪ ▪ ▪

Choose grapefruit heavy for its size. That means it's juicier. It should be shiny and firm, yet give slightly when pressed. Stay away from dull, pebbled, or airy fruit.

You can leave grapefruit at room temperature for up to a week or keep it in the refrigerator for two weeks. You can also freeze the juice and zest.

A serrated knife can help loosen grapefruit segments. You can also use a grapefruit spoon, which has a serrated tip.

Grapes

■ ■ ■ ■ ■ ■ ■ ■ ■ ■ ■

Old-world fruit still fights disease

Next time you enjoy a glass of wine with dinner, you should propose a toast — to grapes. These tiny fruits with sweet, juicy flesh rank among the world's oldest — and most cultivated — fruit.

They have stood the test of time for a reason. Not only do grapes provide lots of vitamin C and vitamin K, along with copper, potassium, and fiber, they're also chock-full of disease-fighting phytochemicals.

Grapes are used to make jams and jellies, dried to make raisins, and squeezed into grape juice and wine. Studies show this common fruit juice can lower blood pressure and could help fight cancer and boost your brainpower as well. But you don't need to turn grapes into something else to enjoy them. Table grapes make delicious snacks.

Grapes come in green, red, or black varieties, with or without seeds. They grow in bunches on climbing vines. California produces nearly all the grapes in the United States, while Italy, France, and Spain rank among the world's leading grape producers. No matter where your grapes come from, they improve your health in a variety ways. Cheers!

Enjoy a "bunch" of benefits for your heart. Grapes come in bunches — and so do their heart-healthy powers. Drinking wine or grape juice can help improve

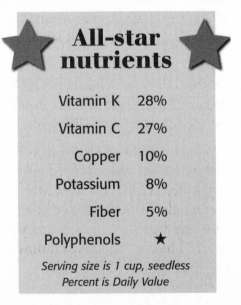

All-star nutrients

Vitamin K	28%
Vitamin C	27%
Copper	10%
Potassium	8%
Fiber	5%
Polyphenols	★

Serving size is 1 cup, seedless
Percent is Daily Value

your cholesterol levels, blood pressure, and blood vessel function. It may even help you live longer.

Researchers have long noticed something called the French Paradox. Despite eating a high-fat diet, the French have low levels of heart problems. But they also drink red wine, which appears to provide protection. And even though alcohol, including wine, tends to raise blood pressure, moderate wine drinkers with high blood pressure have lower death rates.

According to a 40-year Dutch study, people who drank about half a glass of wine a day outlived nondrinkers by an average of four years. Wine drinkers were 46 percent less likely to die of heart problems during the study.

But that's no reason to start drinking alcohol, which comes with its own health risks. You can get similar benefits from grape juice. Studies show that grape juice lowers LDL, or bad cholesterol. It also prevents LDL from becoming oxidized, which makes it more dangerous to your artery walls. Grape juice also boosts HDL, or good cholesterol, and lowers some markers of inflammation, which has emerged as a key risk factor for heart disease.

Other studies have found grape juice lowers blood pressure in people with both high and normal blood pressure. Although the effect was modest, even a small drop in blood pressure can dramatically reduce your risk for stroke and heart-related deaths.

For further proof that something other than the alcohol in wine deserves the credit for its health benefits, another study found that a nonalcoholic grape product improved blood vessel function and even blunted the negative effects of a high-fat meal.

So if it's not the alcohol, what gives wine its power? It could be resveratrol, an antioxidant found in the skin of grapes used to make red wine. While animal studies of resveratrol show much promise, you would likely need to drink an unreasonable amount of wine to reap any benefits. Rather, procyanidins in wine probably help your heart. These condensed tannins are just some of the many phytochemicals found in grapes.

The flavonoids in grape juice increase the production of nitric oxide, which helps relax blood vessels and improve blood vessel function. Purple grape juice has the highest number of proanthocyanidins per serving of any beverage, including red wine, tea, and cranberry juice cocktail. These potent antioxidants could be the secret to grapes' success.

Both purple and red grape juice will protect your heart. If you prefer wine, stick to red wine, which has more antioxidant polyphenols than white wine. Just remember to drink in moderation. That means no more than 4 ounces of wine each day for women and 8 ounces for men.

▪▪▪▪▪ Boost the benefits ▪▪▪▪▪

Your wine glass isn't the only place to take advantage of the health benefits of grapes. Throw some grapes in your salads or add them to creamy sauces or rice dishes. They go well with poultry, wild game, rabbit, fish, and seafood. You can use them in place of apples or cherries in pastries, simmer them to make syrup for pancakes or ice cream, or turn them into jams, jellies, or preserves.

Call on cluster of cancer fighters. Wine may do more than help your heart. A weekly glass of wine may also guard you from colon cancer. One study found that only 1 percent of wine drinkers had significant colorectal polyps, a precursor to colon cancer, compared to 18 percent of beer or liquor drinkers and 12 percent of nondrinkers. Another study found that three or more glasses of red wine a week lessened your risk for colon cancer.

The polyphenols in grapes likely do the trick. A University of Georgia lab study found that the polyphenols from muscadine grapes had anticancer properties. In a University of Illinois lab study, anthocyanin-rich Concord grape extract protected human breast cells from DNA damage. Anthocyanins are antioxidants that give grape juice its deep purple color.

Resveratrol, an antioxidant polyphenol found in grapes, inhibits the growth of several tumor cells, including leukemia, prostate, breast, and liver cells. It also sparks cancer cell death, or apoptosis, in esophageal cancer cells.

Another compound in grapes called pterostilbene, which is similar to resveratrol, may also fight cancer. Pterostilbene prevented cell damage in lab tests using mouse mammary cells. Antioxidants like pterostilbene and resveratrol destroy free radicals, which contribute to cancer. Dark-skinned grapes contain the most pterostilbene. Surprisingly, pterostilbene is not normally found in wine.

Lower your blood sugar to stem diabetes. Pterostilbene, an antioxidant compound found in grapes, can lower blood sugar and fight diabetes. One study showed it could lower blood sugar in rats by 42 percent.

The alcohol and polyphenols in wine may also help with diabetes. In a study of diabetic mice, those who received both alcohol and polyphenols after a meal controlled their blood sugar about as well as normal mice.

An Italian study found that drinking a moderate amount of red wine with meals helps people with diabetes prevent heart complications after a heart attack. Drinking wine before or with your meal can also lower your post-meal blood sugar by up to 37 percent, according to a recent Australian study.

Another study found that women who drank red wine at least once a week had a 16-percent reduced risk of diabetes compared to those drinking wine less than once a week.

Cultivate a healthy brain. Drinking three or more glasses of fruit juice a week could reduce the risk of Alzheimer's by 76 percent compared to people who drink juice less than once a week. Because purple grape juice contains the most polyphenols, it's an excellent choice.

Several animal studies also show grapes may help aging brains. Concord grape juice improved thought processes and body movements in aging rats, while resveratrol added to fish food helped fish live longer and slow age-related declines in memory and motor skills. Cabernet sauvignon and muscadine wines both helped reduce rats' risk of Alzheimer's, and epicatechin, a chemical found in grapes as well as chocolate, tea, and blueberries, improved the memory of mice.

Moderate wine drinking can also have a major impact on your brain's health. In a four-year study of older people, those who drank up to three servings of wine daily reduced their risk for Alzheimer's disease by 45 percent.

Another study found that one drink of wine a day does not impair thinking skills and may actually decrease the risk of mental decline in women.

Red wine protects your brain, thanks to the polyphenol resveratrol. Resveratrol helps by lowering the levels of the amyloid-beta peptides, which cause the plaques found in the brains of Alzheimer's victims.

In spite of these positive study results, health professionals don't recommend you drink alcoholic beverages. The benefits might not outweigh the risks. Talk with your doctor and follow his recommendations.

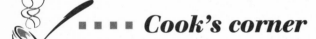

▪ ▪ ▪ ▪ *Cook's corner* ▪ ▪ ▪ ▪

- Seek out plump, firm, fragrant grapes. Avoid soft, wrinkled, shriveled ones. Store them — unwashed — in the refrigerator in a perforated plastic bag for up to 10 days.

- Buy organic grapes when possible because grapes are often treated with chemicals. Rinse well in cold water before serving.

- Remove small clusters of grapes from the main stem with scissors. Don't just pull off individual grapes or the stem will dry out and the other grapes will soften and shrivel.

Honeydew

Sweet melon helps you beat disease

Dr. Bunsen Honeydew, the Muppets' bespectacled yet eyeless mad scientist, did not invent the honeydew. But, if he did, this tasty winter melon would rank among his better inventions.

Honeydew, like all melons, got its start in Africa or India thousands of years ago. Melons, which belong to the same family as the cucumber, squash, watermelon, and gourd, grow on trailing vines in warm climates. Today, most American honeydews come from California.

Slightly more oval than round, honeydew melons usually weigh between 4 and 8 pounds. As they ripen, the color of their smooth outer skin changes from pale green to white to creamy yellow.

With its extremely sweet, light green flesh and soft texture, honeydews can be a treat for your taste buds. With plenty of vitamin C, potassium, folate, vitamin B6, and the carotenoid lutein, honeydew can also be a treat for your body's health.

Put a damper on high blood pressure. Here's an easy way to lower your blood pressure and risk of stroke — boost your potassium intake. This key mineral also helps blunt the effects of sodium on your blood pressure. The best way to get potassium is from food, not supplements. Eating more honeydew, which gives you 388 milligrams of potassium per cup, will help do the trick. Because high blood

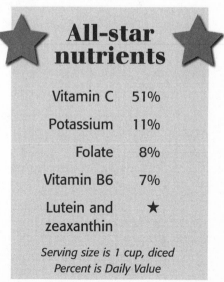

All-star nutrients

Vitamin C	51%
Potassium	11%
Folate	8%
Vitamin B6	7%
Lutein and zeaxanthin	★

Serving size is 1 cup, diced
Percent is Daily Value

pressure is the main risk factor for stroke, honeydew helps prevent stroke, as well. In fact, a potassium-rich diet can reduce the risk of stroke by 22 to 40 percent.

In addition to potassium, honeydew provides lots of vitamin C, which may help lower your blood pressure by keeping your arteries flexible. Honeydew also gives you plenty of folate, a heart-healthy B vitamin that protects your heart by lowering homocysteine levels. High levels of this amino acid may boost your risk of heart attack and stroke.

▪ ▪ ▪ ▪ ▪ Boost the benefits ▪ ▪ ▪ ▪ ▪

Honeydew tastes great as it is, but you can jazz it up by flavoring it with ginger or lemon or lime juice. You can also find several ways to fit honeydew into your diet.

Add honeydew to cereals, fruit salads, cold soups, or smoothies. In fact, a hollowed-out honeydew half makes a great container for fruit salads or cold soups.

Honeydew also goes especially well with ham, deli meats, prosciutto and other dried meats, smoked fish, and cheese. You can also skewer some honeydew as an edible garnish for beverages.

Say goodbye to kidney stones. Potassium does more than just regulate your blood pressure. As an added bonus, the potassium from fruits and vegetables like honeydew also helps fight kidney stones. Potassium helps reduce the amount of calcium excreted in the urine, which also reduces the risk of kidney stones. Studies show that a high potassium and magnesium intake, from a diet rich in fruits and vegetables, can reduce kidney stone formation by up to 50 percent.

Discover the secret to sturdy bones. Honeydew may be soft, but that doesn't make it wimpy. In fact, with its potassium and vitamin C, honeydew can help strengthen your bones.

Potassium guards against osteoporosis the same way it prevents kidney stones — by reducing the amount of calcium excreted in the urine. In fact, a recent study of postmenopausal women found that potassium helps counteract the calcium loss associated with a high-salt diet. By retaining more calcium, you boost your bone strength.

Vitamin C also plays a key role in bone formation. It helps certain enzymes work properly and is essential in the cross-linking of collagen fibers in bone. Getting more vitamin C into your diet, perhaps by eating more honeydew, can improve your bone health.

Cut down on cataracts. Without good eyesight, you wouldn't be able to appreciate the beauty of a honeydew melon. Luckily, eating honeydew keeps your eyes in tip-top shape.

Low levels of vitamin C in the lens of your eye may boost your risk for cataracts. Getting more vitamin C, a common antioxidant, into your diet may help. One study, conducted in Spain, found that higher blood levels of vitamin C lowered the risk for cataracts by 64 percent. A recent Japanese study also found that a higher intake of dietary vitamin C leads to a reduced risk for cataracts.

Honeydew also contains the carotenoids lutein and zeaxanthin, which may protect you from cataracts and macular degeneration. People with cataracts often have a deficiency of these antioxidant carotenoids. Several studies show eating more foods high in lutein and zeaxanthin lowers your risk of developing cataracts or requiring surgery to remove them.

Watch out for little-known allergy

If you are allergic to ragweed, you may want to avoid honeydew, which is a cousin of this wild weed. Honeydew may trigger some of the same symptoms, including sneezing, coughing, congestion, runny nose, headaches, and irritated eyes.

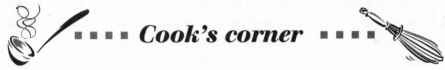

..... *Cook's corner* .....

Choose honeydew that's heavy for its size, without any bruises or cracks. It should give to gentle pressure. A truly ripe melon will feel sticky and give off a honey aroma.

You can let honeydew ripen at room temperature for four days. If you refrigerate melons, whether cut or uncut, make sure to wrap them tightly in plastic because they absorb odors of other foods.

Always buy melons whole. Exposure to air diminishes their nutrient content. So stay away from halves, quarters, or cubes.

Kiwi

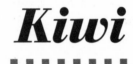

Soar to better health with an unusual fruit

Named for the hairy, flightless national bird of New Zealand, the kiwi may fly under the radar in your local produce section. But you'd have to be a birdbrain to overlook this unusual fruit.

About the size and shape of a large hen's egg, the kiwi has a hairy, dull-brown skin. Inside, it sports emerald green flesh, with rows of black, edible seeds. These seeds give kiwi a texture similar to a strawberry. Kiwi tastes like a blend of strawberry, pineapple, and sweet melon. It also provides a powerful blend of important nutrients, such as vitamin C, vitamin K, fiber, potassium, vitamin E, and copper.

Kiwis, which grow on large, woody vines, got their start in China. In fact, they were once called Chinese gooseberries. In 1906, seeds arrived in New Zealand, where the fruit got its new name. California started growing kiwi commercially in the 1960s. The United States also imports kiwi — now officially known as kiwifruit — from Chile and New Zealand.

While the kiwi bird may not get off the ground, kiwifruit can help your health soar to new heights.

Tasty way to thwart blood clots. You probably know taking aspirin daily helps prevent blood clots, which can lead to heart attack or stroke. But you can also protect yourself with a safer and tastier option — kiwi.

In a study conducted by the University of Oslo in Norway, people who ate two or three kiwifruit a day for a month significantly lowered their risk of developing blood clots. They also slashed their levels of harmful triglycerides by 15 percent. Researchers remain unsure why kiwi helps, but its vitamin C, vitamin E, and polyphenols could all contribute. Vitamin C may help prevent clogged arteries and high blood pressure, while vitamin E serves as a natural blood thinner that may stop the formation of clots. Kiwi also provides plenty of heart-healthy fiber and potassium, which helps control your blood pressure.

Brightly colored fruit safeguards your vision. With its hairy exterior and bright green flesh, kiwi can certainly catch your eye. It can also protect your eyesight.

That's because it's loaded with vitamin C. This antioxidant vitamin may help prevent cataracts and works with other antioxidants — like vitamin E — to slow the progression of

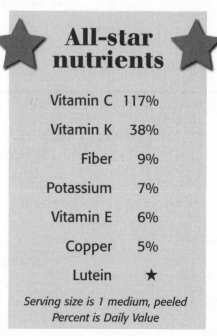

All-star nutrients

Vitamin C	117%
Vitamin K	38%
Fiber	9%
Potassium	7%
Vitamin E	6%
Copper	5%
Lutein	★

Serving size is 1 medium, peeled
Percent is Daily Value

age-related macular degeneration. Vitamin E may also help improve your vision if you have glaucoma.

In addition to antioxidant vitamins, kiwis contain a substantial amount of lutein. This carotenoid plays a key role in guarding your eyes from cataracts and macular degeneration.

■ ■ ■ ■ ■ **Boost the benefits** ■ ■ ■ ■ ■

Kiwi tastes great by itself, but it can also spruce up several other foods. Slices of kiwifruit brighten up your fruit salads, while kiwi wedges can garnish any meal.

Serve a spicy kiwi salsa over meat or add kiwi to fish, poultry, or meat dishes. Kiwi also goes well with avocado, radicchio, and endive. For a refreshing drink, combine fresh kiwi puree, orange juice, and sparkling water.

You can also use kiwi in pies, puddings, and breads. For an exotic dessert, try topping your ice cream with kiwi sauce or slices.

Conquer constipation with a natural remedy. With age comes wisdom. Unfortunately, age often comes with constipation, too. Instead of relying on over-the-counter laxatives, try adding kiwifruit to your diet.

A New Zealand study of 38 healthy people over age 60 found that eating kiwi for three weeks led to easier and more frequent bowel movements. They also had bulkier, softer stools.

The fiber in kiwi likely deserves the credit. While any increase in fiber can help fight constipation, kiwi's fiber may have special properties. The cell walls of kiwis swell considerably during ripening, suggesting that the fiber in kiwi has a high water-holding capacity. This would lead to bulkier stools and improved bowel function. Other kiwi components, including the enzyme actinidin and oligosaccharides, may also play a role.

Silence a wheeze with ease. When it comes to asthma, vitamin C gets an "A." An Italian study of 18,737 children uncovered a positive effect of fruits rich in vitamin C on symptoms of asthma. Children who ate five to seven kiwis or citrus fruits per week reduced their risk for wheezing by 34 percent compared to kids who ate fruit less than once a week. They also fared better in terms of shortness of breath and nighttime or chronic coughing.

Other studies have also found vitamin C beneficial for asthma. It may help because it acts as a natural antihistamine, anti-inflammatory, and antioxidant. A diet low in vitamin C is a risk factor for asthma.

Vitamin C can also come in handy when you're battling a cold. Studies show that high doses of vitamin C may lessen the duration of colds by 5 to 50 percent.

Kiwi is an excellent source of vitamin C. Just one medium-size fruit provides a whopping 70.5 milligrams, or 117 percent of the recommended Daily Value.

■ ■ ■ ■ *Cook's corner* ■ ■ ■ ■

- Look for plump fruit that gives slightly to gentle pressure. Avoid spotted, moldy, or mushy kiwis. You can let unripe kiwi ripen for a few days at room temperature. Speed up the process by putting it in a paper bag with an apple or banana. Refrigerate ripe kiwi in a plastic bag for a week or two.

- Kiwi's fuzzy skin is actually edible, but rarely appealing. Cut off both tips and remove the skin with a vegetable peeler.

- Thanks to an enzyme called actinidin, kiwi can tenderize meat. Just place slices of kiwi on the meat or rub it with the fruit. The same enzyme makes milk curdle and prevents gelatin from setting.

Limes

■ ■ ■ ■ ■ ■ ■ ■ ■

Small citrus fruit puts the squeeze on disease

It's easy to add more zing to your life with limes. Although they are too tart to bite into, these small, green citrus fruits add flavor to other foods. They also help fight disease, thanks mostly to vitamin C. To ward off scurvy, British sailors loaded their ships with limes, earning the nickname "limeys."

Like sailors, limes have done quite a bit of traveling. They probably originated in Asia, around India, Burma, and Malaysia. During the Crusades, they made their way to Europe. Christopher Columbus brought them all the way to America.

Today, southern Florida produces 85 percent of North American limes. Other big lime producers include Mexico, the West Indies, Africa, India, Spain, and Italy. Limes are a basic cooking ingredient in several regions, including Latin America, the West Indies, Africa, India, Southeast Asia, and the Pacific Islands.

Limes, close relatives of lemons, come in two main types — Persian, or common limes, and Key limes, which are smaller and slightly sweeter. In addition to vitamin C, limes provide fiber and small amounts of calcium, iron, and copper.

Amazing way to fight cancer. As a good source of vitamin C, limes are also good weapons against cancer. A new Johns Hopkins University study shed light on how vitamin C may fight cancer. Conventional wisdom says vitamin C scavenges free radicals, which cause DNA damage. But in this latest study,

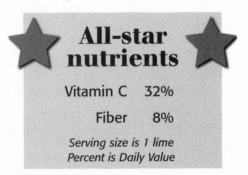

All-star nutrients

Vitamin C 32%

Fiber 8%

Serving size is 1 lime
Percent is Daily Value

cancer cells not treated with vitamin C didn't show any significant DNA damage. They did contain high levels of a protein called hypoxia-inducible factor (HIF-1), while those treated with vitamin C had none.

HIF-1, which depends on free radicals for its survival, helps keep tumor cells alive by helping them compensate for a lack of oxygen. By blocking free radicals, vitamin C slashes HIF-1 levels, indirectly cutting down on tumors.

Limonoids, compounds that give limes and other citrus fruits their bitter taste, have shown anti-cancer promise in animal studies. Limonene, a phytochemical found in the zest of limes, may also help prevent cancer.

A recent Harvard study found that high intakes of citrus fruits, citrus fruit juices, and vitamin C-rich fruits and vegetables helped reduce the risk of oral cancer by 30 to 40 percent.

■ ■ ■ ■ ■ Boost the benefits ■ ■ ■ ■ ■

You know about Key lime pie and margaritas. But limes can play a much bigger — and healthier — role in your diet.

Drizzle lime juice on salad instead of high-fat salad dressing. Sprinkle lime juice on tropical fruit, like mango, papaya, or pineapple, to prevent discoloration and perk up the flavor. Or squeeze some on broiled fish, lamb chops, or steaks.

If a recipe calls for lemons, you can usually use limes instead. The minced zest or juice of limes goes well in soups, sauces, vinaigrettes, ice cream, and sorbets. It can add zing to soft drinks and punches.

Lime juice can act as a meat tenderizer and even "cooks" seafood in ceviche, a classic Peruvian dish of raw fish marinated in lime juice.

Beware of dangerous drug interaction

Limes go great with many foods, but they don't always mix with medication. Like grapefruit, limes may interact with some prescription drugs, leading to a higher than usual concentration of the drug in your bloodstream. In fact, Japanese researchers advise people to avoid any citrus juice when taking medication. Ask your doctor or pharmacist if you should stay away from limes.

Guard your gums from disease. Rearrange the letters in "limes" and you get "smile." That's fitting because limes give your mouth plenty to smile about.

One of the symptoms of scurvy, caused by a vitamin C deficiency, is bleeding gums. Gums can also become swollen, purple, and spongy. Sailors sucked on limes to stave off this condition.

While you probably don't need to worry about scurvy, you should be concerned with periodontal disease, which occurs when bacteria affect the gum and bones that anchor your teeth. Gingivitis and periodontitis, a more advanced form of gum disease, are both forms of periodontal disease. They're also both very common. About half of the United States population has gingivitis while approximately a third has periodontitis.

Getting more vitamin C into your diet can help. A powerful killer of oral bacteria, vitamin C also helps repair connective tissue in your gums. One lime gives you 19.5 mg of vitamin C, or 32 percent of the recommended Daily Value.

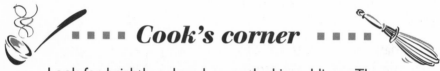

▪ ▪ ▪ ▪ *Cook's corner* ▪ ▪ ▪ ▪

Look for brightly colored, smooth-skinned limes. They should be heavy for their size, but not feel too hard when squeezed. Don't worry about small brown areas on the skin. They won't affect the flavor. But avoid limes with hard or shriveled skin or signs of mold.

You can keep limes at room temperature for about a week or refrigerate them in a plastic bag for up to 10 days. Tightly wrap cut limes in plastic and refrigerate for five days. Scrub with soap and water if you're using the zest.

To get more juice from a lime, roll it firmly between your hands or on the countertop for a minute, then pop it in the microwave for 30 seconds. You can also use your kitchen tongs when squeezing out the juice.

Nectarines

Slick way to triumph over disease

Nectarines look like peaches without the fuzz. While they are about the same size, shape, and color as peaches, their flesh is firmer, and they taste sweeter. The flesh of a nectarine may be white or yellow, with tinges of red close to the pit, or stone.

Native to China, nectarines belong to the rose family. They get their name from the Greek word nektar, meaning "sweet liquid."

Today, 98 percent of the domestic nectarine crop grows in California. The United States also imports some nectarines from South America and the Middle East. Every

All-star nutrients

Vitamin C	13%
Fiber	10%
Vitamin A	9%
Niacin	8%
Potassium	8%

Serving size is 1 medium
Percent is Daily Value

173

once in a while, a peach tree will produce a few smooth nectarines —
and vice versa.

With plenty of vitamin C, vitamin A, fiber, potassium, and
niacin, nectarines provide more than sweet taste. They also provide
some sweet health benefits.

■ ■ ■ ■ ■ Boost the benefits ■ ■ ■ ■ ■

Nectarines make wonderful snacks. Just biting into a
sweet, juicy nectarine can thrill your taste buds. But you
don't have to eat nectarines raw. You can also cook
them. In fact, cooking softens the fruit and really brings
out its sweetness. Bake, grill, broil, poach, or sauté nectarines for a different — and delicious — take on these
sweet treats. You can also substitute nectarines in any
recipe that calls for peaches or apricots.

Shield your eyes with antioxidant vitamins. Look at a nectarine,
and you'll notice its lovely colors. If you want to keep appreciating
those golden and red hues, keep eating nectarines.

Because they provide vitamin C and vitamin A, nectarines may also
provide protection against vision problems. By scavenging dangerous
free radicals that can damage your eye's lens and retina, these antioxidant
vitamins protect your eyes from macular degeneration and cataracts.

Lutein and zeaxanthin, two important carotenoids found in nectarines, also safeguard your eyesight from these common disorders.

While studies involving antioxidant supplements have had mixed
results, adding more colorful fruits, like nectarines, to your diet may
help reduce the risk of cataracts and macular degeneration.

Fortify your heart with flavorful fruit. Nectarines may be small, but
they cram a big dose of heart-healthy nutrients into each delicious bite.
Besides great taste, here's what you — and your heart — get when you
eat a nectarine.

- *Fiber.* One medium nectarine gives you 2.4 grams of dietary fiber. Eating more fiber can lower your blood pressure and slash your risk of heart disease and stroke. Soluble fiber can also lower your cholesterol.

- *Potassium.* This important mineral helps keep your blood pressure under control — especially when you also cut back on sodium. Luckily, a nectarine gives you 285 milligrams of potassium and no sodium. A potassium-rich diet can also protect you from stroke.

- *Vitamin C.* By keeping your blood vessels flexible, vitamin C can help lower your blood pressure. You get 7.7 milligrams of vitamin C in a nectarine.

- *Niacin.* Doctors sometimes prescribe large doses of this B vitamin to raise helpful HDL cholesterol levels. It boosts HDL by up to 30 percent, while also lowering harmful LDL cholesterol and triglycerides. A nectarine provides 1.6 milligrams of niacin — and none of the potential side effects that come with high doses of the vitamin.

■ ■ ■ ■ *Cook's corner* ■ ■ ■ ■

Look for fragrant, plump nectarines that are firm, but not too hard. Ripe nectarines will give to gentle pressure along the seam. They will not be as soft as a ripe peach.

You can put slightly unripe nectarines in a paper bag to speed up their ripening. Refrigerate ripe fruit up to five days. But you should avoid very unripe fruit. If the nectarine has a greenish color, it was picked too early and may not ripen properly. Once picked, a nectarine's sugar content does not increase. Stay away from hard, shriveled, or soft fruits or those with spots, cracks, or bruises.

Buy organic nectarines when possible because nectarines — and peaches — are among the fruits most likely to have pesticide residue.

Olives

■ ■ ■ ■ ■ ■ ■ ■ ■

Change your oil for a longer, healthier life

Jeanne Louise Calment, a Frenchwoman who lived to the ripe old age of 122, credited her longevity to a diet rich in olive oil. That's not surprising. With all the health benefits that come with this tasty oil, it's a wonder she's not still alive today.

This healthy oil lowers cholesterol and blood pressure, fights diabetes, and helps you lose weight. Plus, it lubricates your system, relieving the discomfort of constipation, naturally.

Olives, like Calment, have spent a lot of time on earth. One of the oldest cultivated fruits, olives likely got their start in ancient Greece. Spanish explorers brought them to Peru, and Franciscan monks later carried them to Mexico and California. Today, olive trees thrive in mild climates, such as Mediterranean countries and California.

Not all olives are pressed into olive oil. You can also find a wide variety of table olives, which can be green, red, yellow, tan, brown, or black. Each olive contains a hard pit. Olives provide iron, copper, fiber, vitamin E, and calcium. Fresh olives also contain bitter tannins, so all olives must be processed or cured. Because of this, olives are also high in sodium.

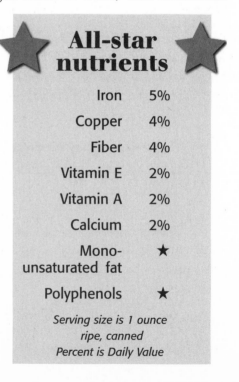

All-star nutrients

Iron	5%
Copper	4%
Fiber	4%
Vitamin E	2%
Vitamin A	2%
Calcium	2%
Mono-unsaturated fat	★
Polyphenols	★

Serving size is 1 ounce ripe, canned
Percent is Daily Value

With olives and olive oil, you get more than great taste. You also get health benefits that last a lifetime — in some cases, an incredibly long lifetime.

Friendly fat lowers cholesterol. "Fat" only has three letters, but for many health-conscious eaters, it's a four-letter word. Olive oil is high in fat — just one tablespoon provides 13 grams of fat. But keep in mind most of that fat is monounsaturated. In fact, olive oil is one of the best sources of this heart-healthy fat.

When you replace less healthy fats, like saturated fat, with monounsaturated fat, you lower bad LDL cholesterol and boost levels of good HDL cholesterol.

Besides monounsaturated fat, olive oil is chock-full of antioxidant compounds called polyphenols. A Greek study found that the polyphenols, vitamin E, and other compounds in olive oil all counteracted LDL oxidation. If you can prevent LDL particles from becoming oxidized, they can do less damage to your arteries.

Olive oil is a key part of the Mediterranean diet, which likely explains the low rates of heart disease in Mediterranean countries. Consider making it a key part of your diet as well.

Natural way to lower blood pressure. Olive oil may not be cheap, but it's a bargain compared to prescription blood pressure medication. It's also much tastier — and almost as effective.

In an Italian study, people who added olive oil to their diet significantly lowered their blood pressure compared to those who added sunflower oil. Better yet, their blood pressure improved so much they were able to cut their daily dosage of blood pressure medication nearly in half. In some cases, they could stop taking it entirely. Researchers suspect the polyphenols in olive oil do the trick.

According to a Spanish study, polyphenol-rich olive oil can also help prevent blood clots. Like high blood pressure, clotting contributes to strokes and heart attacks.

You won't get the same blood pressure benefits from eating olives out of the jar. Because of their high sodium content — just one ounce of olives provides 10 percent of the Daily Value for sodium — olives may not be a good idea if you're trying to control your blood pressure.

■ ■ ■ ■ ■ **Boost the benefits** ■ ■ ■ ■ ■

To get the most from your olive oil, choose the extra-virgin variety, which has the most antioxidant polyphenols. Don't be fooled by light olive oil — the "light" refers to the fragrance and color, not the calories. All olive oil is equally high in fat and calories, so don't go overboard.

Use olive oil for salad dressing, dipping bread, or sautéing. Cooking diced tomatoes with olive oil helps your body absorb more lycopene from the tomatoes.

Olive oil also works as a mild laxative. So if you're feeling constipated, you might just need a quick oil change.

Keep cancer at bay with a powerful weapon. Add more olive oil to your diet, and you may lessen your risk for cancer. In fact, one study estimated that if Western countries adopted the Mediterranean diet — which includes more fruits and vegetables, less meat, and more olive oil — they could prevent up to 25 percent of colon cancers, 15 percent of breast cancers, and about 10 percent of prostate, pancreatic, and endometrial cancers.

Other studies also support olive oil as an anti-cancer weapon. Olive oil consumption lowered breast cancer risk in Spain and Greece. A recent study found that oleic acid, the main form of monounsaturated fat in olive oil, blocks a certain cancer-causing gene. It also increased the effectiveness of a common breast cancer drug.

The polyphenols in olive oil also play a key role in cancer prevention because they scavenge harmful free radicals. Polyphenols from olive oil stopped colon cancer from developing and spreading in lab tests. Olive oil consumption may help prevent colon cancer, according to data from 28 countries and four continents.

A recent Spanish study found that olive oil's polyphenols have a strong antibacterial effect on *Helicobacter pylori*, which has been linked to ulcers and some forms of stomach cancer. The polyphenols even worked against certain strains of the bacteria resistant to antibiotics.

Fight diabetes the tasty way. Olive oil adds flavor to any meal. It also adds several benefits for people with diabetes. You already know how monounsaturated fat, like olive oil, helps lower harmful LDL cholesterol and boost good HDL cholesterol. But olive oil may also improve insulin and blood sugar levels.

Though it packs about 120 calories into each tablespoon, olive oil may also help you lose weight. That's because it fills you up more than other oils. If you're less hungry, you're less likely to snack, overeat, and put on extra pounds. Because olive oil has such a rich flavor, you also don't need to use as much of it.

Natural painkiller soothes arthritis. Whether you cook, dip, or drizzle, olive oil makes your pain fizzle. In a Greek study, people who consumed the most olive oil slashed their risk of developing rheumatoid arthritis by 61 percent compared to those who ate the least. Other studies have shown olive oil relieves arthritis symptoms. Olive oil's monounsaturated fat may fight inflammation or its antioxidants may help by neutralizing free radicals.

But a recently discovered substance in olive oil — a compound called oleocanthal — may also explain the connection. Oleocanthal acts as a natural anti-inflammatory and is very similar to ibuprofen. Inflammation contributes to several health conditions, including rheumatoid arthritis, heart disease, stroke, certain cancers, and some types of dementia.

▪ ▪ ▪ ▪ *Cook's corner* ▪ ▪ ▪ ▪

You can store unopened cans or jars of olives at room temperature for up to two years. Cover loose olives or opened cans with plastic wrap and refrigerate for up to two weeks.

If sealed tightly, olive oil will keep for up to two months at room temperature. Keep it in an opaque, airtight glass bottle or metal tin, away from light and heat. You can refrigerate olive oil for longer. It will become cloudy, but the cloudiness will clear once it returns to room temperature.

Papaya

▪ ▪ ▪ ▪ ▪ ▪ ▪ ▪ ▪ ▪ ▪

Explore exotic fruit and discover super health

Christopher Columbus once called papayas "fruit of the angels." But you don't need a halo and wings to enjoy this heavenly tropical fruit.

Papayas grow on plants that look like trees but are actually over-grown herbs. Native to southern Mexico and Central America, papayas are now mainly cultivated in Hawaii, Mexico, Puerto Rico, and Brazil.

There are two main types of papayas — Hawaiian and Mexican. The Hawaiian, or Solo, papaya weighs about one pound. Its skin turns yellow when ripe, and the flesh can be bright orange or pink. Mexican papayas can weigh up to 10 pounds and have green skin and flesh ranging from red to bright orange. Papayas have a sweet, musky taste and a center full of black, edible seeds that have a peppery flavor.

These large, pear-shaped fruits do more than thrill your taste buds. They also provide plenty of important nutrients, especially vitamin C. You also get vitamin A, folate, fiber, potassium, and vitamin E, as well as vitamin K, magnesium, and calcium in each delicious bite.

Multi-talented enzyme eases indigestion. Next time you feel bloated or gassy after a meal, try a tried and true tropical folk remedy — papaya.

Papaya can help soothe your upset stomach. That's because it contains papain, a unique enzyme that helps break down proteins. Papain is abundant in unripe papayas but fades away as the fruit matures. Once the papaya ripens, only small amounts of the enzyme remain. When the fruit is ready to eat, it has just enough papain to gently boost your digestive process.

You can buy chewable papaya tablets to treat or prevent indigestion, but a glass of unsweetened papaya juice or a wedge of fresh papaya should also do the trick.

The fiber and papain in papayas can also help soothe the uncomfortable symptoms of irritable bowel syndrome. If you suffer from IBS, make room in your diet for papayas.

Nutrients gang up on heart disease. The flesh of the papaya is soft, but this fruit is no softy when it comes to your heart's health. Papayas come packed with nutrients that fight heart disease.

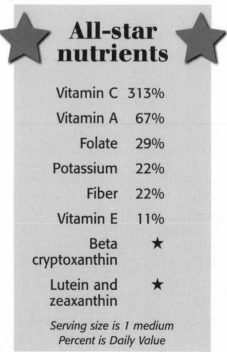

All-star nutrients

Vitamin C	313%
Vitamin A	67%
Folate	29%
Potassium	22%
Fiber	22%
Vitamin E	11%
Beta cryptoxanthin	★
Lutein and zeaxanthin	★

Serving size is 1 medium
Percent is Daily Value

- *Antioxidants.* Loaded with vitamin C, papayas also contain vitamin E and beta-carotene. These antioxidants can prevent bad LDL cholesterol from becoming oxidized. Oxidized LDL sticks to artery walls and forms dangerous plaques that can lead to heart attacks or strokes. Vitamin C may also help fight high blood pressure by keeping arteries flexible.

- *Potassium.* This important mineral helps keep your blood pressure under control. It also helps lower your risk of stroke. A medium papaya has 781 milligrams of potassium, nearly twice as much as a medium banana.

- *Fiber.* From lowering cholesterol to slashing your risk of heart disease and stroke, fiber makes key contributions to heart health. With 5.5 grams of fiber, papaya provides plenty of protection.

- *Folate.* This B vitamin helps counteract a substance called homocysteine, which can damage blood vessel walls and is a major risk factor for heart attack and stroke.

■ ■ ■ ■ ■ Boost the benefits ■ ■ ■ ■ ■

Most people discard the papaya's black seeds. But you can add them to salad dressings for a peppery flavor or even use the seeds in place of black peppercorns.

The rest of the papaya also has plenty of uses. Blend papaya with milk, yogurt, or orange juice to make a delicious shake. Add papaya to fruit salad, salsa, or ice cream or make some refreshing papaya juice. You can always just eat a papaya like a melon. A splash of lime juice really brings out the flavor.

Get creative. Serve cottage cheese, yogurt, ice cream, or chicken or shrimp salad in a hollowed-out papaya.

Stymie cancer with super fruit. Papaya may come from the tropics — but not the Tropic of Cancer. That's because this tropical fruit has several cancer-fighting components.

> ## *Beware of blood thinners*
>
> You may want to avoid papaya if you're taking warfarin or other blood-thinning drugs. The papain in papaya can increase the effects of these medications.

Rich in fiber, papaya guards against colon cancer. The fiber binds to cancer-causing toxins in the colon to shield them from healthy colon cells. Other nutrients in papaya, including vitamin C, vitamin E, beta carotene, and folate, have also been linked to a reduced risk of colon cancer.

Folate also provides protection against pancreatic cancer. In a recent Swedish study, women who got at least 350 micrograms (mcg) of folate from food each day cut their risk for pancreatic cancer by 75 percent compared to those who got less than 200 mcg. One medium papaya gives you 116 mcg of folate.

Eye-opening boost for your vision. If you want to protect your eyesight, then set your sights on papayas. Low levels of vitamin C have been linked to the development of cataracts. Luckily, you'll have no shortage of vitamin C when you add papaya to your diet. With 188 milligrams of vitamin C, papayas provide a whopping 313 percent of the recommended Daily Value.

Vitamin E, another antioxidant vitamin in papayas, may help your vision if you have glaucoma. Combined with other antioxidants, like vitamin C, and zinc, it can also slow the progression of macular degeneration.

Papayas also contain lutein and zeaxanthin. These carotenoids play a key role in protecting your eyes from both macular degeneration and cataracts.

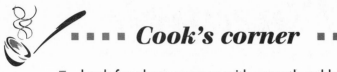

- Look for plump papayas with smooth, unblemished skin. They should be yellow and give very slightly to pressure. Stay away from hard, shriveled, or mushy fruit. Also, avoid papayas with dark spots, which often go beneath the surface and ruin the flavor.

- Ripen papayas at room temperature for three to five days. You can put a papaya in a paper bag with a banana to speed the ripening process. Refrigerate ripe fruit for up to three days.

- Papaya makes a great meat tenderizer, thanks to the enzyme papain, which breaks down tough meat fibers. Papain works so well that it is an ingredient in some commercial powdered meat tenderizers. Add some papaya to your marinades.

- You can find another unusual meat tenderizer in your kitchen cabinet — vinegar. Even the most inexpensive meat goes from tough to tender with just a tablespoon of this kitchen staple. Just add it to the water before boiling, and you'll be able to cut your stew meat with a fork.

Pineapple

■ ■ ■ ■ ■ ■ ■ ■ ■ ■ ■ ■ ■ ■ ■ ■

Prickly peel hides powerful fruit

Like a soft-hearted dragon, a pineapple is prickly on the outside but sweet on the inside. This large tropical fruit can measure up to a foot in length and weigh up to 10 pounds. Covered in a scaly skin that may be yellow to reddish-brown or green to greenish-brown, pineapple's juicy, fragrant flesh ranges from nearly white to yellow.

Native to southern Brazil and Paraguay, pineapples came to Europe with Christopher Columbus and spread to other parts of the world on ships that carried it to ward off scurvy. The desire to grow pineapple in England sparked the development of the greenhouse.

Today, most pineapples come from Thailand, the Philippines, and Hawaii. They also grow in most tropical regions, including Central and South America, the Caribbean, Australia, the Pacific Islands, and many parts of Asia and Africa.

Pineapples grow on a plant that is technically an herb with large, waxy, pointed leaves. Each pineapple is actually a compound of small individual fruits called "eyes," merged into one large fruit. Its name comes from the Spanish *piña* because Spanish explorers thought it resembled a pine cone.

Don't let its prickly exterior fool you. Inside lurks a wealth of nutrients. Loaded with vitamin C and manganese, pineapple also provides fiber, copper, potassium, magnesium, and several B vitamins.

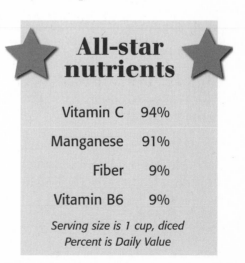

All-star nutrients

Vitamin C	94%
Manganese	91%
Fiber	9%
Vitamin B6	9%

Serving size is 1 cup, diced
Percent is Daily Value

■ ■ ■ ■ ■ **Boost the benefits** ■ ■ ■ ■ ■

Besides eating pineapple raw, you can enjoy it cooked, grilled, broiled, sautéed, or in baked goods.

Just don't mix fresh pineapple with gelatin because the enzyme bromelain prevents it from setting. Boiled or canned pineapple will work because heat breaks down bromelain.

Bromelain also helps tenderize meat and poultry, so consider using fresh pineapple in your marinades. But be careful. Letting the meat marinate too long may make it mushy.

Beat digestive disorders with bromelain. The flesh and stems of fresh pineapples contain an enzyme called bromelain that helps break down protein. This makes it an effective meat tenderizer — and a useful digestive aid.

Several studies suggest bromelain helps maintain regularity and relieve constipation. Some nutritionists think eating just 4 ounces of pineapple a day may be enough to end constipation.

It also helps treat and prevent diarrhea caused by the *E. coli* bacteria. In one study, a dose of bromelain kept more than half of a group of piglets exposed to *E. coli* from developing diarrhea. Among those not treated with bromelain, none escaped diarrhea. In fact, the more of the enzyme a piglet was given, the better its chances of avoiding diarrhea.

Experts think bromelain may pick up the slack for people with celiac disease, helping them digest food and giving their digestive system time to heal.

It may do the same for people with ulcerative colitis. Some doctors report bromelain supplements helped people suffering from mild ulcerative colitis by healing the inflamed mucous membrane lining their colons. Animal studies show it may help heal stomach ulcers, as well.

You can get bromelain from eating fresh pineapple, but not canned or cooked pineapple. It's also available as a dietary supplement.

Breathe easier with better diet. What you eat may determine how well you breathe. A recent British study found a link between asthma and a diet low in vitamin C and manganese.

Luckily, pineapples contain plenty of both of these important nutrients. Just one cup of diced pineapple provides 56.1 milligrams of vitamin C, or 94 percent of the recommended Daily Value. It also gives you 1.8 milligrams of manganese, or 91 percent of the Daily Value.

Other studies have found vitamin C beneficial for asthma. It may help because it acts as a natural antihistamine, anti-inflammatory, and antioxidant. Manganese also has antioxidant properties and protects your lungs from oxidative damage.

Vitamin C can also help when you're battling a cold. Studies show that high doses of vitamin C may shorten the length of colds by 5 to 50 percent.

Bone up on bone health. If you're concerned about developing osteoporosis, you probably already try to include plenty of calcium and vitamin D in your diet. Just don't forget to make room for pineapples, which contain several other nutrients essential to bone health. The two main nutrients in pineapple, vitamin C and manganese, play key roles in keeping your bones strong.

Vitamin C, which is involved in bone formation, helps certain enzymes work properly and is required in the cross-linking of collagen fibers in bone. Manganese also helps enzymes work properly to build strong bones. In one study, women who took manganese along with calcium, copper, and zinc had stronger bones than those who just took calcium.

Pineapples also provide smaller amounts of potassium, copper, and magnesium — nutrients that help increase bone mineral density and prevent bone loss.

Block cancer with mighty molecules. Promising new research suggests pineapples may fight cancer. Scientists isolated two molecules from bromelain taken from crushed pineapple stems.

One molecule, called CCS, blocks a protein called Ras that is defective in about 30 percent of cancers. The other, named CCZ, stimulates your body's immune system to target and kill cancer cells. In lab tests, CCS and CCZ blocked several tumor cells, including breast, lung, colon, ovarian, and melanoma. More research is needed, but pineapples could give you an edge in the fight against cancer.

Pineapples also contain plenty of vitamin C and fiber, both of which are highly recommended for general cancer prevention.

■ ■ ■ ■ *Cook's corner* ■ ■ ■ ■

Look for pineapples with fresh, green leaves and no soft or brown spots. The fruit should be plump, heavy for its size, and slightly soft to the touch. One trick is to tap the pineapple lightly with the palm of your hand. If it sounds muffled, that means it's ripe. If it sounds hollow, it may be dried out.

If you buy a pineapple at room temperature, keep it at room temperature. If you buy it chilled, wrap it in plastic wrap and refrigerate it for up to three days.

You can also freeze pineapple. Just peel it, cut it into chunks, and freeze it on a baking sheet. Once frozen, store the pineapple in an airtight container.

Plantains

■ ■ ■ ■ ■ ■ ■ ■ ■ ■ ■ ■ ■ ■

'Cooking bananas' sizzle with surprising benefits

A plantain is no mere second banana. Plantains, or cooking bananas, provide just as many benefits as their sweeter counterparts.

Like bananas, they grow in bunches on banana trees, which are actually giant herbaceous plants. These long, canoe-shaped fruits have green skin that's thicker than that of a regular banana. As the fruit ripens, the skin turns yellow, then black. The flesh, which is firmer and not as sweet as a banana, remains creamy, yellow, or light pink.

Though they become softer and sweeter as they ripen, you should not eat plantains raw, even when ripe. But you can enjoy these starchy relatives of the banana — which have a texture and flavor similar to a sweet potato — in many ways. In fact, plantains are a dietary staple in several regions, including Africa, India, Malaysia, the West Indies, and South America.

With plenty of fiber and nutrients like vitamin C, vitamin A, potassium, vitamin B6, and magnesium, plantains could be an important part of your diet as well.

Soothe an irritated stomach. Gastritis, or inflammation of your stomach lining, can be a sign of a peptic ulcer. It can also be very painful. Plantains, with the ability to treat and prevent ulcers, may be the key to relief.

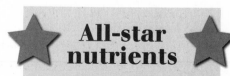

All-star nutrients

Vitamin C	36%
Vitamin A	36%
Potassium	27%
Vitamin B6	24%
Fiber	18%
Magnesium	16%

Serving size is 1 cup, cooked and mashed
Percent is Daily Value

In animal studies, plantains caused the stomach lining to grow. It thickened, actually preventing new ulcers from forming. It also covered over existing ulcers, allowing them to heal — kind of like putting salve on a cut.

Your diet plays an important role in managing gastritis. In addition to avoiding certain foods that may irritate your stomach — like citrus fruits, spicy foods, or fried and fatty foods — you should make room for soothing foods, like plantains. They help ease inflammation and prevent flare-ups.

▪ ▪ ▪ ▪ ▪ Boost the benefits ▪ ▪ ▪ ▪ ▪

Spruce up your side dishes. Take a break from potatoes, and try plantains instead. Just boil and mash these starchy fruits, as you would a potato.

You can add plantains to soups and stews or blend them with apples, sweet potatoes, or squash. Mash ripe plantains and add them to pancake or muffin batter. You can also roast or pan-fry plantains.

Skip kidney stones with key nutrients. Plantains are packed with potassium, magnesium, and vitamin B6, three nutrients that may help fight kidney stones.

Like their close relative bananas, plantains give you plenty of potassium. Just one cup of cooked, mashed plantains provides 930 milligrams of potassium, or 27 percent of the recommended Daily Value. It also contains 64 milligrams of magnesium, or 16 percent of the Daily Value.

Large studies show that getting lots of potassium and magnesium into your diet, through fruits and vegetables, slashes your risk of kidney stones by 30 to 50 percent. Eating more plantains can help.

Plantains are also a good source of vitamin B6, giving you 0.5 milligrams, or 24 percent of the Daily Value. A deficiency in this vitamin can lead to an increase in the production of oxalate, a risk factor for stones. Women who boost their intake of vitamin B6 may reduce their risk of kidney stones.

Solidify your bones with a smart diet. Add plantains to your diet, and you'll add plenty of protection against osteoporosis. With several important vitamins and minerals, plantains can help you dodge brittle bone disease.

Potassium helps preserve calcium in your bones, keeping them strong. Eating more potassium-rich foods, like plantains, can boost hip and forearm bone mineral density in older people.

About 60 percent of the magnesium in your body lies in your bones. This mineral appears to improve bone quality and bone mineral density. Not getting enough magnesium may interfere with your body's ability to process calcium.

Your body needs vitamin C to help enzymes work properly to build strong bones. This antioxidant vitamin also stars in the crosslinking of collagen fibers in bone.

Vitamin B6 does not directly influence bone health, but it may help indirectly because of its effect on vitamin K, which plays a key role in bone metabolism. Interestingly, people with hip fractures get significantly less vitamin B6 in their diet than those without fractures.

Set your sights on saving your vision. Plantains come in many colors. Depending on their level of ripeness, they can be green, yellow, or black. Peel away their colorful outer layer, and plantains give your eyes plenty of other reasons to appreciate them.

That's because plantains contain vitamin A, vitamin C, and the carotenoids lutein and zeaxanthin — nutrients that protect your eyesight.

Low levels of vitamins A and C can lead to cataracts, while vitamin C — in combination with other antioxidants and zinc — can also help slow the development of macular degeneration. Lutein and zeaxanthin, powerful antioxidants your body stores in the retina of your eyes, help prevent cataracts and macular degeneration.

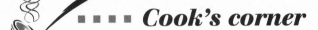

Cook's corner

Choose plump, unblemished plantains at any stage from green to black. Remember, brown or black skin does not affect the quality of the flesh. It just indicates ripeness.

Keep plantains at room temperature. They may take up to two weeks to ripen — but you can cook with plantains at any time.

You can store very ripe plantains in the refrigerator for about a week. You can also freeze them. Just peel and wrap them individually.

Plums

The inside story on a misunderstood fruit

Little Jack Horner, of nursery rhyme fame, got quite a present when he used his thumb to pull a plum from his Christmas pie. Packed with antioxidants, fresh plums provide vitamin C, vitamin A, vitamin K, fiber, and potassium. Dried plums, also known as prunes, have a higher concentration of fiber and minerals, but little vitamin C.

Plums come in several shapes, sizes, and colors. They can be as small as a cherry or as big as a baseball, and their skin can be yellow, green, red, blue, purple, or almost black. Their juicy flesh ranges from red or orange to yellow or greenish yellow and has a sweet and tart balance. As a drupe, or a fruit with a single pit, the plum is related to the peach, nectarine, and apricot.

First cultivated in China, plums were also appreciated by ancient Egyptians, Etruscans, Greeks, and Romans. Today, plums grow mainly in Russia, China, Romania, and the United States. Most U.S. plums — and nearly all of the prunes — come from California. Michigan and New York also grow some plums.

Eat them fresh or dried — or even pull them from a pie. No matter how you enjoy plums, you'll get plenty of health benefits.

Conquer constipation with dried plums. If dried plums are famous for anything, it's their ability to keep you regular. These wrinkled treats overcome constipation in a number of ways.

Much of the credit goes to their high fiber content. A dozen dried plums provide about 7 grams of dietary fiber, which helps speed your stool through your system.

Besides fiber, dried plums also contain sorbitol, a sugar alcohol that acts as a natural laxative. That's probably why prune juice, which has no fiber, also helps relieve constipation.

Fresh plums also provide fiber and sorbitol, but both substances are more concentrated in dried plums. Antioxidant polyphenols in dried plums may also contribute to their laxative action.

Adding dried plums to your diet can help keep your digestive system running smoothly. Just make sure to drink plenty of water, too.

Chewy snack prevents brittle bones. Preventing osteoporosis could be as simple as snacking on dried plums. In an Oklahoma State University study, postmenopausal women who ate 12 dried plums a day for three months had higher levels of insulin-like growth factor-1

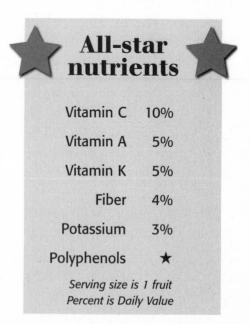

All-star nutrients

Vitamin C	10%
Vitamin A	5%
Vitamin K	5%
Fiber	4%
Potassium	3%
Polyphenols	★

Serving size is 1 fruit
Percent is Daily Value

(IGF-1) and bone-specific alkaline phosphatase activity — two key markers of bone formation.

Researchers speculate that antioxidant polyphenols in prunes led to the improvement in bone health, but the trace elements boron and selenium also play a role in preserving bone mineral density.

Several other nutrients make prunes a good weapon against osteoporosis. A dozen prunes contains a whopping 74 percent of the Daily Value of vitamin K, which may improve bone mineral density and reduce your risk of fractures. Dried plums also give you plenty of potassium, manganese, copper, and magnesium, which all contribute to better bone health.

Previous studies have shown prunes help reverse bone loss in rats, and a current Florida State University study is exploring whether they do the same for women with osteoporosis.

■ ■ ■ ■ ■ Boost the benefits ■ ■ ■ ■ ■

Trim the fat from your cakes and brownies. Pureed prunes make a good substitute for butter, oil, or other fats in baked goods. It's a good way to add moisture and fiber without any fat. You can find dried plum puree, or prune butter, in the baking aisle or near the jams and jellies at the supermarket.

You can also add chopped plums to fruit salads, broil or grill them with chicken or fish, or cook them with pork or game. They can even replace fresh cherries in most desserts.

Pleasant way to keep cancer at bay. Dried plums may not look like much, but these little fruits may help you avoid cancer. In a recent Japanese laboratory study, an extract taken from concentrated prune juice blocked human colon cancer cells and triggered apoptosis, or cell death. The prune extract did not affect healthy colon cells.

Prunes are also rich in fiber and antioxidants, which can help prevent cancer. Experts recommend eating more fruit to prevent all types of cancers, so fill up on both fresh and dried plums for maximum protection.

Sidestep dangerous food poisoning. Prunes not only taste good, they can also make your food safer to eat. A recent Kansas State University study showed that prune puree and fresh plum juice concentrate kill certain strains of bacteria that cause food poisoning. For example, just one tablespoon of prune puree per pound of ground beef can kill more than 90 percent of *E. coli*.

The antioxidant phenolic compounds in prunes, including neochlorogenic acid and chlorogenic acid, do the trick. The prune mixtures also worked against *Salmonella* and *Listeria*.

Of course, you still want to cook your meat thoroughly to guard against food poisoning. But adding some prune puree to your ground beef could make your burgers a little safer — and tastier.

▪ ▪ ▪ ▪ *Cook's corner* ▪ ▪ ▪ ▪

Choose plump, firm plums with a pleasant scent. They should yield to slight pressure of the fingers — but do not squeeze them. Stay away from plums that are too soft or too hard. Avoid those with cracks, bruises, blemishes, or stains.

Let plums ripen at room temperature, and store ripe plums in your refrigerator for a few days. You can also freeze plums, but you should remove the pit first so the flesh doesn't become bitter.

Pomegranate

■■■■■■■■■■■■■■■■■■■■

Sow the seeds of good health

Though only the pomegranate's seeds and juice are edible, there are many great reasons to try this unusual fruit. Among fruits, pomegranate has the highest level of antioxidants — those incredible tumor and blood clot fighters. It also provides plenty of vitamin C and potassium. This luscious fruit can protect your vision, battle heart disease, save your memory, release you from arthritis pain, and more.

Pomegranates are large, round fruits with leathery skin ranging from red to yellowish pink. Inside, you'll find hundreds of small, ruby-red seeds covered in a juicy pulp. The seeds are packed into compartments separated by a bitter membrane. The seeds taste great, leaving you with a refreshing feeling in your mouth and throat. The membrane and skin are inedible.

Native to Persia, pomegranates grow on a dense shrub that can reach 12 feet in height. Today, they grow in the Middle East, Africa, India, Malaysia, southern Europe, and the United States — chiefly California, where the Wonderful variety is most common.

One of seven fruits to appear in the Old Testament, the pomegranate has long been a symbol of fertility. On the other hand, the hand grenade got its name from the pomegranate because of its similar size and seed-like shrapnel.

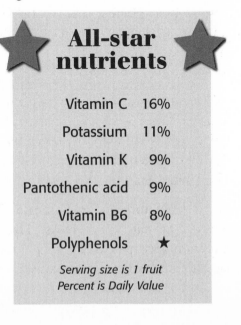

All-star nutrients

Vitamin C	16%
Potassium	11%
Vitamin K	9%
Pantothenic acid	9%
Vitamin B6	8%
Polyphenols	★

Serving size is 1 fruit
Percent is Daily Value

Pomegranate translates to "apple or fruit of many seeds," but it could just as easily mean "fruit of many health benefits."

Hammer heart disease with antioxidants. Just as each pomegranate contains hundreds of small seeds, this fruit is also loaded with powerful antioxidants that fight heart disease.

Several studies involving both people and mice show that pomegranate juice helps combat atherosclerosis, or hardening of the arteries. The antioxidant polyphenols in pomegranate juice stop oxidation of LDL, or bad cholesterol. Once LDL becomes oxidized, it becomes more dangerous to your artery walls. Polyphenols' antioxidant activity stymies the development of fatty deposits that form inside your artery walls. These fatty deposits can rupture and block blood flow, leading to heart attack or stroke.

Even if you already have heart disease, pomegranate juice can help. In one study, people with heart disease who drank pomegranate juice for three months showed a 17-percent improvement in blood flow to the heart. Those in the control group, who drank a modified sports drink instead, worsened by 18 percent.

As a bonus, pomegranate juice helps prevent atherosclerosis in people with diabetes. And despite being high in sugar, the juice does not worsen blood sugar. That's because the sugars are attached to unique antioxidants, which actually make the sugars protective against atherosclerosis. In a small Iranian study, pomegranate juice even lowered total and LDL cholesterol in people with diabetes.

Prevent prostate cancer with polyphenols. Real men drink pomegranate juice — or at least they should. That's because pomegranate juice comes packed with polyphenols that protect you from prostate cancer, the second leading cause of cancer-related death among men in the United States.

In laboratory studies, pomegranate extracts showed no mercy against human prostate cancer cells. Thanks to their antioxidant and anti-inflammatory properties, they inhibited cell growth, slowed tumor growth, and triggered apoptosis, or cell death.

■ ■ ■ ■ ■ **Boost the benefits** ■ ■ ■ ■ ■

Brighten up your salads, soups, oatmeal, meat dishes, and desserts with pomegranate seeds. Much more than a garnish, the seeds add texture, color, and a welcome burst of flavor to your food.

Mix pomegranate juice with lemonade for a refreshing drink. Or use the juice to make syrup for sundaes or savory sauces.

One home remedy for upset stomach and diarrhea involves drinking tea made from pomegranate skin. The skin contains tannins, which relieve stomach irritation by helping your body produce a mucous lining in your stomach.

A UCLA study found that drinking a daily 8-ounce glass of pomegranate juice significantly slows the increase in prostate-specific antigen, or PSA — an indicator of cancer. The researchers measured "doubling time," or how long it takes for PSA levels to double. Men with short doubling times are more likely to die from cancer. In the study, which involved men who had been treated for prostate cancer, PSA doubling times increased from an average of 15 months to an average of 54 months.

Ellagitannins, the most abundant polyphenols in pomegranate juice, get much of the credit for the juice's anti-cancer powers.

Avoid arthritis with anti-inflammatory fruit. Protect your joints with pomegranate. Researchers recently discovered a new way this ancient fruit can improve your health.

When you have osteoarthritis, you need to worry about a substance called Interleukin-1b (IL-1b). This troublemaker creates an excess of inflammatory molecules, including matrix metalloproteases (MMPs), which break down cartilage, leading to joint damage and destruction.

In lab tests of human cartilage cells, pomegranate fruit extract stopped the overproduction of MMPs, protecting the cartilage from the damaging effects of IL-1b.

Known for its antioxidant and anti-inflammatory powers, pomegranate could be a weapon against osteoarthritis.

Give your memory a boost. When it comes to avoiding Alzheimer's disease, remember pomegranate juice. Loma Linda University researchers made an important discovery recently. Mice that drank pomegranate juice had about 50 percent less brain degeneration than those who got sugar water. They also learned water maze tasks more quickly and swam faster than the other mice as they aged.

The high concentration of antioxidants in pomegranate juice helps protect your brain from damaging free radicals. Drinking a glass or two of this healthy beverage a day just might save your memory.

See fewer eye problems with vitamin C. As a good source of vitamin C, pomegranates can help you avoid common vision problems.

Studies suggest vitamin C can prevent cataracts. Getting more of this antioxidant vitamin into your diet can lower your risk of developing cataracts or lessen your need for cataract surgery. High levels of vitamin C in your blood can cut your risk of cataracts by 64 percent. On the other hand, low levels of vitamin C in the lens of the eye may lead to cataracts.

Combined with other nutrients, vitamin C can also slow the progression of age-related macular degeneration (AMD). In one study, a diet rich in vitamin C — along with zinc, vitamin E, and beta carotene — reduced the risk of developing AMD by 35 percent.

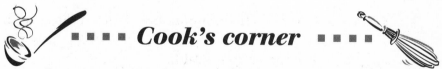

■ ■ ■ ■ *Cook's corner* ■ ■ ■ ■

Pomegranates can be messy. Minimize the splatters and stains by removing the seeds in a bowl of water. First, cut a pomegranate into quarters. Fill a bowl with cold water, and hold each pomegranate quarter under the water seed side down. Use your fingers to scoop out the seeds, which will sink to the bottom of the bowl. The bitter pieces of membrane will float to the top, where you can easily gather and discard them. Drain the seeds and pat them dry with a paper towel.

To get at the juice, roll a pomegranate on a hard surface while pressing it with the palm of your hand. This will release the juice from the seeds. Then make a small hole, insert a straw, and sip. Or squeeze the fruit over a glass. You can also buy pomegranate juice at the supermarket.

Raspberries

Gamble on brambles to beat disease

Comparing another fruit to a raspberry seems like a mismatch. After all, the raspberry has the other fruit outnumbered. That's because each raspberry is actually made up of several individual fruits, each with its own seed, surrounding a central core. These tiny, hairy fruits, or "drupelets," cling to one another like a close-knit family.

Like blackberries, which are smooth and hairless, raspberries are considered brambles. They come in two main varieties — black raspberries, with their purplish black flesh, and the more common red raspberries. Both kinds are fragrant and sweet, with a slightly tart taste.

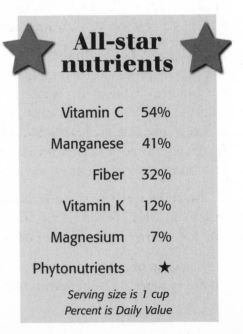

All-star nutrients

Vitamin C	54%
Manganese	41%
Fiber	32%
Vitamin K	12%
Magnesium	7%
Phytonutrients	★

Serving size is 1 cup
Percent is Daily Value

200

Brimming with phytonutrients, raspberries also provide plenty of vitamin C, manganese, and fiber. No wonder they were used medicinally hundreds of years ago.

Leading producers of these disease-fighting fruits include Russia, Poland, Germany, Chile, and the United States. Red raspberries thrive in the Pacific Northwest, while black raspberries pop up in the eastern United States and Canada. Make sure raspberries also pop up in your diet, and these little powerhouses will gang up on health problems.

Eat to beat cancer. If you're worried about cancer, it's a good idea to eat more fruit. It's an even better idea to make sure some of those fruits are raspberries.

An Ohio State University study of rats found that raspberries helped fight colon cancer. Scientists infected rats with colon cancer and fed some of them black raspberries. The rats developed 80 percent fewer cancerous tumors than those kept on a regular diet.

Researchers credit the abundance of antioxidants in raspberries for their success. Anthocyanins, which give berries their color, phenols, and vitamins could all contribute to raspberries' ability to fight cancer. Even among antioxidant-rich berries, raspberries stand out. Black raspberries have 11 percent more antioxidant activity than blueberries and 40 percent more than strawberries.

Ellagic acid, a phenolic compound found in red raspberries, has also shown promising anti-cancer potential. In lab tests conducted at the Hollings Cancer Institute at the University of South Carolina, ellagic acid stopped cell division and triggered apoptosis, or cell death, in breast, pancreatic, esophageal, skin, colon, and prostate cancer cells. As a good source of fiber and vitamin C, raspberries provide even more protection against cancer.

No sweat way to save your bones. Raspberries tingle your taste buds with their sweet and subtly tart flavor. They also give your bones a thrill with key nutrients that prevent osteoporosis.

Eat a cup of raspberries, and you'll get 32.2 milligrams of vitamin C. That's 54 percent of the recommended Daily Value. Your body needs vitamin C to help certain enzymes work to build strong bones and for the cross-linking of collagen fibers in bone.

■ ■ ■ ■ ■ **Boost the benefits** ■ ■ ■ ■ ■

Sick of strawberries? Try raspberries instead. They are interchangeable with strawberries in most recipes. You can also find several ways to fit more of them in your diet.

Top your ice cream or yogurt with raspberries. Garnish fruit salads, cereals, cakes, and crepes. Puree raspberries to create dessert sauces or tasty beverages. You can also make them into syrups, jams, or jellies.

Blend raspberries with olive oil and balsamic vinegar to make a delicious raspberry vinaigrette for your salad. For a refreshing drink on a hot day, add frozen raspberries to your lemonade in place of ice cubes.

Like vitamin C, manganese helps enzymes work better to build strong bones. Combined with calcium, copper, and zinc, it can lead to a greater increase in bone compared to calcium by itself in women who are postmenopausal. You'll get 0.8 milligrams of manganese, or 41 percent of the Daily Value, in a cup of fresh raspberries.

That same cup of raspberries gives you 9.6 micrograms of vitamin K, or 12 percent of the Daily Value. Low levels of this important vitamin may mean lower bone mineral density and higher risk of fracture. Raspberries also contain smaller amounts of magnesium, copper, potassium, iron, phosphorus, zinc, and calcium — minerals essential to bone health.

Foil constipation with a fabulous fruit. Snack on raspberries, and stop struggling with constipation. Just one cup of raspberries packs a whopping 8 grams of fiber, or 32 percent of the recommended Daily Value. Fiber adds bulk to your stool and helps speed it through your digestive system. Adding fiber-rich foods, like raspberries, to your diet can help keep you regular. Just make sure to drink plenty of water, as well.

You don't even have to eat the fruit of the raspberry bush to benefit from it. Raspberry leaves are an herbal remedy for diarrhea and other intestinal disorders, including upset stomach, nausea, and vomiting. Steep two teaspoons of raspberry leaves in boiling water for a soothing tea you can drink up to three times a day — but do n't overdo it. Stronger brews may actually provoke nausea and diarrhea in some people.

While little research exists to explain why this age-old remedy works, scientists have some clues. The leaves are rich in tannins, which have astringent qualities that are helpful for diarrhea. Their soluble pectin fiber and flavonoids also contribute to good overall intestinal health.

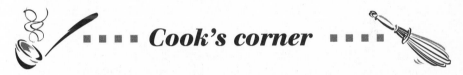

■ ■ ■ ■ *Cook's corner* ■ ■ ■ ■

- Choose plump, firm, round, bright berries, and avoid those with dents or bruises. Turn the container over to look for stains, a sign of overripe or decaying berries. You should also gently shake the container to uncover any insects that may be hiding in there.

- Raspberries are among the fruits most likely to have high levels of pesticide residue, so buy organic when possible. If you pick your own berries, pick ripe ones, since they don't ripen after picking. For sweeter, longer-lasting berries, pick them in the morning.

- Raspberries are very perishable. Keep them in the refrigerator, where they will last a day or two. Don't wash them until just before serving.

Rhubarb

Fruit-like veggie 'stalks' disease

A loud argument is sometimes called a rhubarb. But there's no reason to get into a rhubarb over rhubarb, despite this plant's confusing classification.

While technically a vegetable, rhubarb is used as a fruit. Except for its pink color, this tart relative of buckwheat and sorrel looks like celery. Only its long, pink stalks, which can be 1 to 3 inches thick, are edible. Loaded with vitamin K, rhubarb also provides plenty of vitamin C, manganese, calcium, potassium, and fiber.

As far back as 2700 B.C., the Chinese used rhubarb for medicinal purposes. Marco Polo brought rhubarb to Europe around 1200, but Europeans did not commonly use it for food until the late 1700s. When it made its way to the United States soon afterward, rhubarb earned the nickname "pie plant" because it was a popular filling for pies. Today, rhubarb plants — perennials that can reach more than 3 feet high — grow throughout Oregon, Washington, and Michigan.

The name "rhubarb" means "root of the barbarians" in Latin, with the term "barbarian" referring to anything unfamiliar or foreign. Rhubarb may be unfamiliar to you, but there are plenty of reasons to make this fruity vegetable a part of your diet.

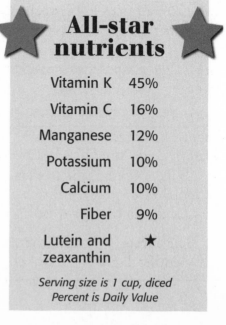

All-star nutrients

Vitamin K	45%
Vitamin C	16%
Manganese	12%
Potassium	10%
Calcium	10%
Fiber	9%
Lutein and zeaxanthin	★

Serving size is 1 cup, diced
Percent is Daily Value

■ ■ ■ ■ ■ **Boost the benefits** ■ ■ ■ ■ ■

While rhubarb is too tart to eat raw, you can still enjoy it. Just thinly slice the stalks, then bake or stew them, and add some sweetener. Rhubarb becomes sweeter with cooking, so wait until after cooking to add sugar, honey, or maple syrup. Mixing rhubarb with sweet fruit, like strawberries, is a good way to cut down on sweetener — and calories.

Rhubarb also goes well with apples, blueberries, raspberries, apricots, and raisins. Use it in savory dishes, pair it with meats and fish, or make a rhubarb sauce to top your pancakes, waffles, or French toast. You can also season rhubarb with lemon, cinnamon, and ginger.

Give your digestive system a nudge. Prized for its laxative action for centuries, rhubarb still helps relieve constipation. It also stops diarrhea and aids in digestion.

Although a good source of fiber, rhubarb gets most of its digestive benefits from its phytochemicals. Phenols called anthraquinone glycosides, which give rhubarb stalks their red color, act as a natural laxative. They are the same compounds found in other laxative herbs, like cascara and senna. The tannins in rhubarb, on the other hand, help stop diarrhea.

Rhubarb benefits digestion from the moment it enters your mouth. It stimulates your taste buds with its pleasantly bitter flavor, making your mouth feel clean and refreshed. Once it reaches your stomach, rhubarb's digestive benefits really kick in — stimulating the production of gastric juices and improving digestion. It also helps control the absorption of fat in your intestines.

The effects of rhubarb root extract have received lots of attention in scientific literature. Low doses seem to relieve diarrhea, while higher doses help keep you regular. But before you head to the herb shop, consider this — the same phytochemicals contained in the roots are found in smaller amounts in the edible stalks. Plus, you'll get vitamins, minerals, and fiber not found in the extract.

Cool hot flashes with ease. You may want to change your diet to deal with your "change of life." Rhubarb may hold the key to handling menopause.

During perimenopause, the transitional stage before menopause when women experience irregular menstrual cycles, you may also deal with hot flashes, sweating, sleep disturbances, and mood swings.

A 12-week German study of 109 perimenopausal women found that an extract from rhubarb root, given in pill form, helped ease their symptoms. They experienced fewer and less severe hot flashes and improved their quality of life. The extract, called ERr 731, does not contain estrogens, and researchers remain unclear how it works.

While you may not get the same benefit from rhubarb, this vegetable does provide other nutrients important to older women, including vitamin K, potassium, and manganese, which are essential to bone health. It's also a good source of calcium, although oxalate prevents your body from absorbing much of it. You also get vitamin C and the carotenoids lutein and zeaxanthin, which protect your eyes from macular degeneration and cataracts.

Leave rhubarb leaves alone

Never eat rhubarb leaves. Their high levels of oxalates make them toxic. You could experience weakness, burning in the mouth or throat, difficulty breathing, abdominal pain, nausea, vomiting, and diarrhea. You could even die, although you would need to eat a large amount of leaves.

Although stalks contain safer amounts of oxalates, these compounds can contribute to kidney stone formation. Your doctor may recommend avoiding or limiting rhubarb if you're prone to kidney stones.

Protect your pancreas in an unusual way. As an unusual vegetable, it's only fitting that rhubarb helps fight an unusual condition called pancreatitis.

Pancreatitis means inflammation of the pancreas. When you have this condition, digestive enzymes produced by the pancreas become active within the pancreas rather than the small intestine. That means the pancreas starts to attack, or digest, itself.

This can be a life-threatening illness with many complications. It begins with pain in the upper abdomen, which can extend to the back and other areas. You may also experience nausea, vomiting, fever, and rapid pulse. Severe cases lead to organ failure, shock, and even death.

Rhubarb has helped alleviate the seriousness of the first stages of pancreatitis, while preventing complications in later stages. In a recent Chinese study involving rats, researchers found rhubarb had protective effects on severe acute pancreatitis. Rhubarb probably works by fighting inflammation, improving circulation in the small blood vessels of the pancreas, and inhibiting pancreatic enzyme. Of course, you still need to seek medical care for serious attacks. But rhubarb may be a helpful addition to standard treatment.

▪ ▪ ▪ ▪ *Cook's corner* ▪ ▪ ▪ ▪

Look for firm, crisp rhubarb with deep red stalks. Throw away the leaves, then store the stalks in the refrigerator. Rhubarb wilts quickly, so use it within a few days. Trim both ends of the stalk. You may want to peel off the tough outer skin, too.

You can also buy rhubarb frozen or canned. If you want to freeze your own rhubarb, stew it, blanch it, or sweeten it with sugar first.

When cooking rhubarb, do not use a cast iron or aluminum pan. The acids in rhubarb will react with the metal and leave both your pan and your rhubarb blackened.

Starfruit

Wish upon a starfruit for better health

All fruits are stars when it comes to nutrition, but only the starfruit really looks the part. These oval fruits have a shiny, waxy surface and greenish yellow skin with five prominent pleats, or ribs, that run along the length of the fruit. When you cut a starfruit crosswise, you end up with slices shaped like five-pointed stars, which give the fruit its name.

With light to dark-yellow, crispy, juicy flesh, starfruit tastes like a blend of grape, plum, and tart apple. Each fruit comes with up to 12 small, tender, edible seeds. It also comes with plenty of vitamin C and fiber, as well as copper, potassium, and pantothenic acid, or vitamin B5.

Also known as the carambola, starfruit got its start in Sri Lanka or Malaysia and has been cultivated in Southeast Asia for centuries. Around 1887, it made its way to Florida. Later, it popped up in Hawaii. Today, it grows in Taiwan, Malaysia, Guyana, India, the Philippines, Australia, Israel, Brazil, China, and the United States.

Try this unusual star-shaped fruit, and discover a galaxy of health benefits.

Fistful of nutrients guards your heart. Each slice of starfruit has five points. It also has five mighty nutrients that protect your heart. Just imagine each point — and each nutrient — as a finger. United, they can form a fist to clobber heart disease.

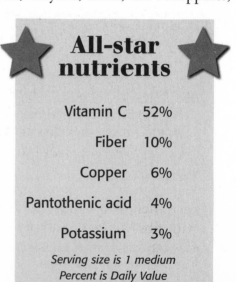

All-star nutrients

Vitamin C	52%
Fiber	10%
Copper	6%
Pantothenic acid	4%
Potassium	3%

Serving size is 1 medium
Percent is Daily Value

- *Vitamin C.* This antioxidant vitamin has a helpful effect on blood pressure because it keeps arteries flexible.

- *Fiber.* Getting more fiber into your diet helps lower your risk of heart attack and stroke. Soluble fiber can lower cholesterol.

- *Copper.* A deficiency of this mineral may lead to high cholesterol, heart disease, high blood pressure, irregular heartbeat, and heart attack. By promoting the growth of new blood vessels, copper helps offset damaging stress. This amazing mineral can also prevent an overworked heart from enlarging.

- *Potassium.* This key mineral helps regulate blood pressure and reduces your risk of stroke.

- *Pantothenic acid.* This B vitamin, also known as vitamin B5, plays a key role in the metabolism of food and production of essential body chemicals. A derivative of pantothenic acid, called pantethine, may lower cholesterol and triglycerides.

■ ■ ■ ■ ■ **Boost the benefits** ■ ■ ■ ■ ■

Add flair — and nutrition — to any dish with a garnish of starfruit slices. Replace lemon slices with starfruit slices for fish or seafood dishes. Garnish iced tea, tropical drinks, appetizers, cheese platters, or desserts with starfruit.

Throw some starfruit into your fruit salad, even though it might "outshine" the other fruits. You can also grill it on skewers with shrimp or chicken, stir-fry it with seafood and vegetables, or puree it for chutney, sauces, soups, and jams. Use it for marinades or make it into a refreshing juice.

Strengthen your bones with starfruit. It's only fitting that a fruit with ribs can help protect your bones. Starfruit contains nutrients that can ward off osteoporosis.

When to say no to starfruit

If you have kidney failure, stay away from starfruit. You run the risk of suffering from starfruit intoxication. Symptoms include persistent hiccups, vomiting, mental confusion, weakness, numbness in your limbs, insomnia, and seizures. In some cases, your blood pressure may drop, and you could go into shock or even die.

Vitamin C helps certain enzymes work better to build strong bones. It also plays a key role in the cross-linking of collagen fibers in bone. Older women can raise their bone mineral density with this important vitamin.

Two minerals found in starfruit, potassium and copper, also boost your bone health. Potassium helps your bones retain much-needed calcium. It also improves bone mineral density in women making the transition to menopause. In older people, it boosts the bone mineral density in hips and forearms.

Copper deficiency decreases bone strength in animals, while copper supplementation reduces bone loss in older women. That's because this mineral affects bone formation and the strength of your connective tissue.

Antioxidants help you see the light. There's nothing quite as majestic as gazing at the stars. To appreciate every twinkle, just turn your gaze to starfruit. With antioxidants like vitamin C, beta-carotene, and lutein and zeaxanthin, starfruit helps safeguard your vision.

Low levels of vitamin C in the lens of your eyes can lead to cataracts. Fortunately, getting more of this vitamin into your diet can help you avoid cataracts and cataract surgery. One medium starfruit gives you 31.3 milligrams of vitamin C, or 52 percent of the recommended Daily Value.

When combined with other antioxidants, including beta-carotene, vitamin C can help slow the progression of macular degeneration, the leading cause of blindness in older people.

Lutein and zeaxanthin, carotenoids that act as powerful antioxidants, shield your eyes from macular degeneration and cataracts.

Studies show eating more foods with lutein and zeaxanthin can slash your risk for macular degeneration by 57 percent and lower your risk for cataract surgery by 22 percent.

■ ■ ■ ■ *Cook's corner* ■ ■ ■ ■

Choose firm, shiny starfruit with a pleasant scent. Avoid those with blemishes or soft spots. Handle with care because they bruise easily. Most tart varieties have very narrow ribs, while the sweet yellow kinds have thick, fleshy ones.

Let starfruit ripen at room temperature until it becomes solid yellow. You can refrigerate ripe fruit in the refrigerator for a week or two. Use a vegetable peeler or paring knife to remove the tips of the ribs if they turn brown or black.

Tangerines

■ ■ ■ ■ ■ ■ ■ ■ ■ ■ ■ ■ ■ ■ ■ ■ ■ ■

Enjoy easy-to-peel, ready-to-heal citrus fruit

Mandarin oranges got their name because their rind was the same color as the robes worn by mandarins, or Chinese public officials. One important type of mandarin orange, the tangerine, is still serving the public.

Packed with vitamin C, vitamin A, fiber, potassium, and folate, tangerines keep you healthy in several ways. One extra serving a day of this mouth-watering fruit can reduce strokes, lower obesity, and fight heart disease.

Smaller than oranges, tangerines appear slightly flattened. Their thin, red-orange rind peels easily, revealing segments of juicy flesh. Less acidic than most citrus fruits, tangerines taste sweet with a hint of tartness. They are the most nutritious of all mandarins, which also include clementines and tangelos.

Native to China, tangerines now grow all over the world on ever-greens that reach about 10 feet. Tangerines get their name from the ancient, walled Moorish town of Tangier in northern Morocco, where the fruit thrives. Most tangerines in the United States come from California, Arizona, and Florida.

In some parts of the world, tangerines are a traditional Christmas or New Year's treat. But you don't need to wait for a special occasion to enjoy these delicious and healthy fruits.

Slash stroke risk with citrus. Tangerines may be small, but they can make a big difference against heart disease and stroke. Like other citrus fruits, they contain an unbeatable combination of nutrients, including phytonutrients, that help your heart.

The potassium in citrus fruits, like tangerines, lowers blood pressure just like pills. A British study found that potassium citrate, the type of potassium in fruits and vegetables, works just as well as potassium chloride, the type sometimes prescribed for lowering blood pressure. As a bonus, getting potassium from foods rather than pills eliminates the risk of side effects.

Speaking of risks, a large study found that one extra serving of citrus fruit a day reduced the risk of stroke by 19 percent. Drinking extra citrus juice helped even more, lowering the risk by 25 percent.

Other studies have found that vitamin C helps fight heart disease. Just one serving of vitamin C-rich fruits and vegetables

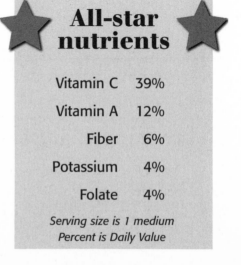

All-star nutrients

Vitamin C	39%
Vitamin A	12%
Fiber	6%
Potassium	4%
Folate	4%

Serving size is 1 medium
Percent is Daily Value

a day can lower your risk by 6 percent. The folate, fiber, and flavonoids in tangerines and other citrus fruits also contribute to better heart health.

▪ ▪ ▪ ▪ ▪ Boost the benefits ▪ ▪ ▪ ▪ ▪

Tangerines make great snacks. But you can find several other ways to make the most of these healthy fruits. Add them to green salads or fruit salads, dip them in yogurt, or substitute them for oranges in recipes.

Don't forget about the juice and the zest. Drink the refreshing juice by itself or blend it with other fruit juices. Pouring tangerine juice over freshly sliced fruit will prevent it from browning and add flavor. You can also make marinades and dressings with the juice. Add tangerine zest to sauces, desserts, and marinades.

Slim down with super fruits. Losing the battle of the bulge? Adding more tangerines to your diet can help. Not only are tangerines very low in calories, they also provide fiber, which fills you up so you don't overeat. Your body can't digest fiber, so it passes through your system. A high-fiber diet can help keep your weight in check.

Eating fruit, like tangerines, on a regular basis can help you avoid weight gain. A 12-year study of thousands of women found that the ones who ate the most fruit were less likely to become obese during middle age. While all citrus fruits are good choices, tangerines may be one of your best bets. They normally contain more water and less sugar than oranges.

Here's more good news. Orange juice may be an effective appetite suppressant — but timing is everything. Have orange juice before dinner, and studies show you'll eat less. Have it with dinner, and you'll gain weight.

In a Yale University study, overweight men who drank orange juice before their meal ate nearly 300 fewer calories at lunch than those who drank plain water. Overweight women consumed an average of 431 fewer midday calories.

However, a Pennsylvania State University study found that women who drank high-calorie beverages, including orange juice, with lunch took in an extra 104 calories without feeling any fuller.

For a surprisingly simple weight loss secret, drink a glass of orange juice a half-hour to an hour before a meal. You'll eat fewer calories during the meal and still feel comfortably full. Stick to plain water with meals.

Boost your defense against cancer. When it comes to cancer prevention, a healthy diet is essential. Tangerines can be an important part of any anti-cancer eating plan.

A laboratory study found that pectin, a type of complex carbohydrate found in citrus fruits, helps fight prostate cancer. Of the fruits tested, tangerines had the most pectin. To get the most of pectin, eat the whole fruit, not just the juice. The flesh of the fruit and the membranes that separate the segments contain the highest concentration of pectin.

Cryptoxanthin, a carotenoid abundant in orange fruits like tangerines, may reduce your risk of cervical cancer. A molecule called salvestrol Q40, found in the peel of tangerines, also has shown promise as a cancer fighter.

Several studies show that citrus fruits can protect against cancer, especially oral and stomach cancers. In one study, high intakes of citrus fruits and juices lowered the risk of oral premalignant lesions by 30 to 40 percent.

Catch your breath with vitamin C. Tangerines may be a breath of fresh air in your struggle with asthma. A yearlong Italian study found that citrus fruits, including tangerines, had a protective effect against asthma symptoms. Children who ate five to seven citrus fruits a week lowered their risk of wheezing by 34 percent compared to kids who ate fruit less than once a week. They also fared better in terms of shortness of breath and nighttime or chronic coughing.

The vitamin C in citrus fruits probably provides protection. It may help because it acts as a natural antihistamine, anti-inflammatory, and antioxidant. A diet low in vitamin C is a risk factor for asthma.

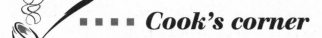

Cook's corner

If you're impatient, tangerines are the fruit for you. They're always picked ripe, so you can eat them right away.

Look for firm, shiny tangerines that are heavy for their size. Avoid those with bruises, soft spots, or dents. Medium tangerines are usually best. Very large ones have less taste and very small ones may be bitter.

Store tangerines at room temperature for a week or in a plastic bag in the refrigerator for longer. You can freeze tangerine juice.

Watermelon

Sweet summer fruit offers year-round protection

You probably associate watermelon with good times, like summer cookouts or picnics. But these sweet, refreshing fruits also have a serious side that looks after your health.

Watermelon provides vitamin C, vitamin A, potassium, magnesium, and fiber. It's also a great source of the carotenoid lycopene. Of course, as its name suggests, it contains plenty of water. In fact, a whopping 92 percent of a watermelon is water.

Along with squash, pumpkins, and cucumbers, watermelons belong to the gourd family. They can be round, oblong, or spherical and can weigh up to 90 pounds. The thick but fragile rind can be solid, striped, or speckled, while the sweet, crisp flesh is usually red but can also be orange or yellow. Seeds can be black, brown, white, green, yellow, or red.

Watermelons got their start in Africa, where they were prized as a source of portable water. Ancient Egyptian tombs contain pictures of watermelons, which may also be native to North America. Thomas Jefferson grew watermelons at Monticello, and the Confederate army boiled them down to make sugar and molasses during the Civil War.

Today, the world's leading producers include China, Russia, and Turkey. About 50 varieties of watermelon grow in the United States. For good times and good health, try some of them.

Lessen cancer risk with lycopene. When it comes to lycopene, tomatoes and tomato products get most of the attention. But watermelon actually has 40 percent more lycopene than raw tomatoes. That's good news because studies show this carotenoid can help prevent prostate cancer.

In one recent study conducted in China, researchers found that men who got the most lycopene through their diet slashed their risk of prostate cancer by 82 percent compared to those who got the least. Eating more watermelon also helped.

Another study found that men with the highest blood levels of lycopene reduced their risk of prostate cancer by 35 percent compared to those with the lowest levels.

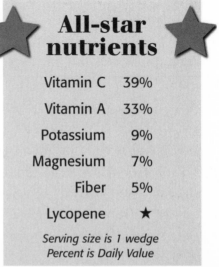

Lycopene, which gives water-melon its red color, acts as an antioxidant, neutralizing free radicals that can cause damage. It may also help protect against other cancers, including those of the breast and pancreas.

Help your heart with a juicy fruit. Bite into a juicy watermelon, and take a bite out of heart disease. Studies show

All-star nutrients

Vitamin C	39%
Vitamin A	33%
Potassium	9%
Magnesium	7%
Fiber	5%
Lycopene	★

Serving size is 1 wedge
Percent is Daily Value

that lycopene, the carotenoid that fights cancer, may also protect your heart.

■ ■ ■ ■ ■ Boost the benefits ■ ■ ■ ■ ■

To get the most out of watermelon, store it at room temperature. It may not be as refreshing, but it will have more nutrients. Compared to freshly picked watermelon, those stored at 70 degrees Fahrenheit have up to 40 percent more lycopene and 139 percent more beta carotene.

Enjoy watermelon in fruit salads or cold soups. Watermelon juice makes a refreshing beverage. To cut down on calories, you can mix it with an equal amount of seltzer. Every part of a watermelon is edible. Pickle the rind or roast the seeds for a tasty snack.

In a Dutch study, older people with high blood levels of lycopene lowered their risk of atherosclerosis, or hardening of the arteries. In another study, Finnish researchers found that men with the lowest levels of lycopene in their blood had thicker carotid arteries, a risk factor for heart attack and stroke. Women with the highest blood levels of lycopene can reduce their risk of heart disease by about one-third compared to those with the lowest levels.

Lycopene's antioxidant powers help stop LDL, or bad cholesterol, from becoming oxidized and forming plaques in your artery walls. Lycopene also helps prevent blood clots in laboratory tests.

Watermelon is also a good source of citrulline, an amino acid your body turns into another amino acid called arginine. As a precursor to nitric oxide, arginine plays a key role in regulating blood pressure and supporting healthy circulation. A U.S. Department of Agriculture study found that drinking watermelon juice boosted blood levels of arginine.

In addition to lycopene and arginine, watermelon also provides potassium, magnesium, and fiber. Potassium and magnesium help control blood pressure, while fiber can lower cholesterol.

Sweet way to lose weight. Here's a fun way to keep your weight under control — eat more watermelon. This tasty fruit can satisfy your sweet tooth without hurting your waistline.

Experts say foods with high water content can help you lose weight. At 92 percent water, watermelon fits the bill. Water fills you up so you're less likely to overeat. It may even boost your metabolic rate, or the rate at which you burn calories.

One slice of watermelon has only about 86 calories and less than half a gram of fat, making it the perfect dessert.

▪ ▪ ▪ ▪ *Cook's corner* ▪ ▪ ▪ ▪

Look for firm, symmetrical melons that feel heavy for their size. Avoid those with bruises, cracks, or soft spots. The underside of the melon should have a yellow spot from where it rested on the ground as it ripened. You can also buy watermelons cut into halves, slices, or quarters. They should smell sweet and have dense flesh.

Keep whole watermelons at room temperature for a week or in the refrigerator up to two weeks. Before slicing a watermelon, scrub the entire outer surface under warm running water to remove surface bacteria. Refrigerate cut watermelon, wrapped in plastic or in an airtight container, and eat it within a few days.

Harvest the goodness of whole grains

Amaranth

■■■■■■■■■■■■■■■■■

New life for an amazing grain

Amaranth may be the most ancient grain you've never heard of. It was a favorite crop of the Aztecs, but it was nearly lost when European conquerors made growing it a crime. The Greeks saw amaranth as a symbol of immortality, and it has enjoyed a rise in popularity during the past 30 years as people seek out more healthy whole grains.

Technically, amaranth isn't really a grain. It's a broadleaf plant with bright flowers and seeds you can eat. Amaranth greens add color and nutrition to salads, and the seeds can be cooked as cereal or used in baking. It packs a wallop when it comes to minerals like manganese, magnesium, phosphorous, and iron, and it's no slouch in the B-vitamins department, either.

Whole-grain foods with lots of fiber are known for helping control your weight, and amaranth certainly has plenty of fiber. But don't over-do amaranth if you're trying to lose a few pounds. The grain is also high in energy, with about 365 calories in a half cup of seeds. That's more than twice the calories in the same amount of oatmeal.

Sidestep celiac disease with gluten-free grain. People with celiac disease, an inherited condition that's also called sprue, are sensitive to the gluten in wheat, barley, and some other grains. The gluten damages their small intestines, making it hard for the body to

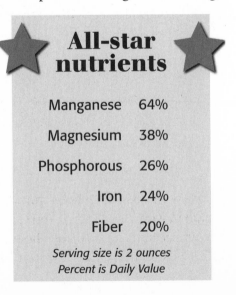

All-star nutrients

Manganese	64%
Magnesium	38%
Phosphorous	26%
Iron	24%
Fiber	20%

Serving size is 2 ounces
Percent is Daily Value

get nutrients from food. The best way to avoid problems is to stay away from gluten. Shunning this ingredient reverses damage to the small intestines in 95 percent of people with celiac disease. But remove all wheat from your plate, and you may be left with little to eat.

That's where amaranth can come to the rescue. It's free of gluten, and it can be a substitute for wheat or other grains. It's available in ready-made dry cereals, and you can buy it as a seed to cook into hot cereal. Boil a cup of seeds in 3 cups of water for about 30 minutes for a hearty, high-protein breakfast that won't damage your digestion.

Amaranth can also be ground into flour and used in baking. It works well in pancakes or cookies, but not in recipes that need to rise, like breads. You can replace up to a quarter of the wheat flour in a bread recipe with amaranth flour to get a moist, nutritious bread. However, gluten from the wheat flour remains.

■ ■ ■ ■ ■ Boost the benefits ■ ■ ■ ■ ■

Popcorn is a whole grain that gets no respect. It's a tasty source of fiber, thiamin, and minerals, so it makes a healthy snack without added butter and salt.

But popcorn is not the only grain with pop. Some types of amaranth seeds can also be popped. Amaranth's nutty, peppery taste, along with its high protein and iron content, make it a healthy treat. Use a wok or heavy skillet for popping. One cup of amaranth pops up into about 3 to 4 cups of delicious snack. Eat it soon as it quickly becomes rancid.

Five ways amaranth helps your heart. Heart disease is a leading cause of death in women and men. You can lower your risk with a heart-healthy diet, which aims to control cholesterol, blood pressure, and weight. Adding this unusual grain to your diet may help you reach these goals.

- Amaranth contains about 6 to 9 percent oil, which one study found lowered total cholesterol, LDL, and triglycerides in people who ate it every day for three weeks. Experts think it's the oil's squalene and phytosterols that keep cholesterol from being absorbed in your intestines. If you want more amaranth oil than is in the grain, look for bottled oil in a natural food store, and use it on salads or in place of other oils.

- The jumbo serving of magnesium in amaranth makes it good for your heart muscle. It boasts 149 grams in 2 ounces of seeds, more than a third of what you need every day. Magnesium helps with more than 300 processes in your body, including keeping your heartbeat regular and helping muscles and nerves work properly. In fact, a four-year study found people who got more magnesium, potassium, and fiber had less risk of high blood pressure. Amaranth has all these and more.

- Amaranth has more protein than other grains, and what it has is a more complete source of the essential amino acids your body needs. That means you can substitute it for some of the meat in your diet, giving you the benefits of muscle-building protein without the saturated fat. Start your day with a bowl of amaranth flakes cereal, and you'll get 6 grams of protein.

- Some research has found that people with celiac disease who followed a gluten-free diet raised their "good" HDL cholesterol levels. That gave them a better balance between HDL and the "bad" LDL cholesterol. Experts think a diet without gluten may heal damaged intestines so you can absorb more HDL. In fact, one study found people with celiac disease who started a gluten-free diet lowered their chances of dying from heart disease.

- With 6 grams of fiber in a 2-ounce serving, amaranth is a whole-grain hit. Fiber — both soluble and insoluble — is important to a heart-healthy diet. It battles high cholesterol, keeps blood pressure in check, helps manage your weight, and lowers your risk of heart disease and diabetes. Heck, it may even fight gum disease and heartburn. How many more reasons do you need to try the high-fiber goodness of amaranth?

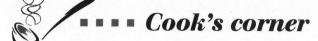

Cook's corner

Use the whole shebang. You can take advantage of the entire amaranth plant since the leaves, stems, and seeds are all edible.

Store parts separately. Keep amaranth flour in a nontransparent container in a cool, dry place. It lasts longer than wheat flour. Store the seeds the same way. You can refrigerate amaranth leaves for a few days, or freeze them as you would spinach.

Enjoy growing amaranth. This hardy plant grows well in many conditions. Its stems and flowers may be purple, orange, red, or gold. Wild varieties with dark seeds make good ornamentals and potted plants. Varieties with pale seeds are better sources of the grain.

Know the difference. Don't confuse the amaranth plant and grain with the amaranth dye, Red dye number 2. It's a man-made dye used on leather, silk, and other products, but it's not from the plant. It was used in foods — including red M&Ms — until the U.S. Food and Drug Administration banned it in 1976.

Brown rice

Enjoy this nutty, nutritious grain

A Chinese proverb says, "Even the cleverest housewife can't cook without rice." That may be true in Asia, where a person may eat up to 400 pounds of rice each year, but not in the United States, where 20 pounds a year is more typical. A cook in the West could go forever without serving rice.

That's a shame, because rice is a cheap dish that goes well with other foods and brings a big bowl of nutrition to the table. Brown rice, the whole rice kernel with only the hull removed, is especially nutritious. It's high in fiber, niacin, and vitamin B6, and it's a great source of minerals like manganese, magnesium, and selenium. Brown rice boasts a sweet, nutty flavor and a richer texture than white rice. Rice is also an important part of the BRAT diet — bananas, rice, applesauce, and toast — which is bland, nutritious, and helpful when you are getting over a bout of diarrhea.

A symbol of fertility, rice is often thrown at weddings to wish the happy couple good luck and many children. Toss a bit more brown rice into your diet to win your own good luck and good health.

Nip colon cancer in the bud. Your choice of white or brown rice may affect whether you get colon cancer. Some studies show eating more fiber — like the 4 grams of fiber in a cup of cooked long-grain brown rice — may lower your chances of developing tumors in your large intestine, or colon.

In fact, rice bran, the part that makes the rice look brown, contains most of the fiber in brown rice. Researchers in England wondered if this fiber might prevent certain tumors. They fed rice bran to mice and checked to see if they developed cancer of the colon, prostate, or breast tissue. The mice that ate lots of rice bran — the equivalent of 200 grams in a human diet — had half the risk of intestinal tumors but no

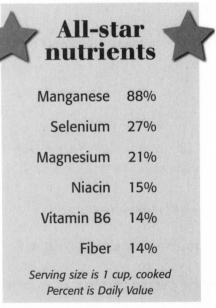

All-star nutrients

Manganese	88%
Selenium	27%
Magnesium	21%
Niacin	15%
Vitamin B6	14%
Fiber	14%

Serving size is 1 cup, cooked
Percent is Daily Value

change in the other cancers. The scientists think the fiber in rice bran is what protected the mice.

But brown rice is also high in vitamin B6, which may also prevent colon cancer. A study of Swedish women found those who took in more vitamin B6 had less chance of getting colon cancer during the 15 years they were followed. Yet another study found people who got more vitamin B6 and folate, another B vitamin, from food had a lower risk of colon cancer.

■ ■ ■ ■ ■ **Boost the benefits** ■ ■ ■ ■ ■

Brown rice is naturally full of nutrients, high in fiber, and low in fat. Keep it healthy by cooking it wisely.

First, don't rinse rice before cooking. If nutrients were sprayed onto rice grains to enrich it, you may wash away that extra goodness. Second, cook rice in water without adding fat. For more low-fat flavor, cook it in vegetable, beef, or chicken stock. Add flavor with herbs or spices like basil, cilantro, or parsley.

Brown rice is available as instant rice, which cooks in just five minutes rather than the usual 45 minutes. It's been precooked and then dried, but this processing makes it less nutritious than regular brown rice.

Control diabetes with stable blood sugar. People with diabetes must watch what they eat to keep a balance between blood sugar and insulin. Foods with a high glycemic index (GI), like white bread or potatoes, make your blood sugar level rise quickly — maybe too fast for your body to handle it. Many doctors urge people with diabetes to focus on foods with a low GI, like whole grains or beans. Brown rice, with its outer layer of bran and fiber, has a GI of 66. That's a better choice than the more refined and polished white rice, which has a GI of 72. More processing into puffed rice cereal pushes the GI all the way up to 90.

In fact, research proves eating more whole grains like brown rice may lower your risk for type 2 diabetes. When researchers examined more than 2,000 people in the Framingham Offspring Study, they found those who ate at least three servings of whole grains each day had less risk of developing metabolic syndrome. This condition is often a warning that diabetes or heart disease may be in your future. Ward off blood sugar woes by choosing fiber-filled brown rice over the more refined white rice.

▪ ▪ ▪ ▪ *Cook's corner* ▪ ▪ ▪ ▪

Get a grip on grains. With more than 8,000 types of rice around, how can you tell the difference? One way is by size. Brown rice comes in three lengths.

- Long-grain rice has grains more than a quarter inch long. It's the most popular type in the United States, and grains tend to stay separate during cooking.

- Medium-grain rice has grains up to a quarter inch long. It keeps more moisture when cooked than long-grain rice.

- Short-grain rice has round grains shorter than one-fifth of an inch long. It tends to be sticky after cooking because it contains more starch.

Don't be fooled by the name. Wild rice is not really rice at all. It's an annual grass in a different cereal family than actual rice. Although wild rice used to be gathered from plants growing wild in lakes, most of it is now planted as a crop. It's not even "wild" anymore.

Pick a plate of wholesome pasta

When it comes to pasta, the ingredients used to make the noodles determine its nutrition. Certain new "healthy" pastas have twice the fiber or protein of traditional pasta. Using soy in pasta adds soy protein and isoflavones, which may help your heart and prevent some diseases. But you may pay more than twice as much to eat well. See how these popular varieties stack up against each other in calories, fiber, and other nutrients.

Pasta (2 oz dry, enriched)	Calories	Fiber	Noteworthy nutrients	Price per ounce
Barilla Plus thin spaghetti	200	4 g	10 g protein 10% iron 15% riboflavin 15% niacin 30% folate 35% thiamin	$.16
Ronzoni Healthy Harvest whole-wheat blend thin spaghetti	180	6 g	6 g protein 10% iron 15% riboflavin 20% niacin 30% folate 35% thiamin	$.16
Revival soy thin spaghetti	200	1 g	14 g protein 15 mg isoflavones 2% calcium 15% iron 15% phosphorous	$.33
Regular pasta	211	2 g	7 g protein 10% iron 13% riboflavin 20% niacin 34% folate 34% thiamin	$.09

Oatmeal

■ ■ ■ ■ ■ ■ ■ ■ ■ ■ ■ ■

Fiber-filled favorite is chock-full of goodness

Known as pilcorn in Merry Old England, oatmeal was a favorite traditional food in Scotland. This beloved comfort food was first planted in the New World in 1602 — when William Shakespeare was busily writing his plays and Queen Elizabeth was lording it over her empire. Oatmeal is now commonly eaten hot and steaming in a bowl at breakfast, but the grain can also be baked into muffins, breads, or cakes and added to meatloaf and pancakes.

Oatmeal gets high marks for fiber, but it also scores in the vitamins-and-minerals department. Whether quick-cooking, regular, or instant, one cup of oatmeal is a good source of the B vitamin thiamin and the minerals manganese, selenium, and phosphorus. It also keeps away hunger until lunchtime — all for a measly 147 calories.

Cut your cholesterol down to size. You've seen the ads. The doting grandfather explains to his grandchild why he's eating oat cereal for breakfast — to get ready for his cholesterol test. Then a fast-talking announcer explains that adding oats to your diet can lower your cholesterol. It sounds simple, and it works.

So how does eating oatmeal help keep your cholesterol goals on track? It's all about the fiber. Oatmeal, along with some other grains like barley, contains beta glucan, a soluble fiber shown to

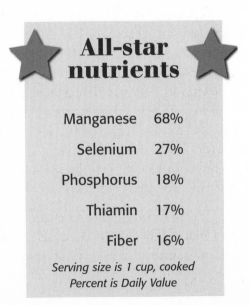

All-star nutrients

Manganese	68%
Selenium	27%
Phosphorus	18%
Thiamin	17%
Fiber	16%

Serving size is 1 cup, cooked
Percent is Daily Value

help lower LDL and total cholesterol. Beta glucan combines with water to form a gel, which slows down food as it moves through your digestive tract. This gives HDL more time to pick up and remove cholesterol from your blood, while LDL has less chance to attach to artery walls. Good work all around.

The link between beta glucan and cholesterol is so clear that the U.S. Food and Drug Administration allows companies to make this claim on products with at least 0.75 grams (g) per serving of whole oats: "Soluble fiber from foods such as oat bran, as part of a diet low in saturated fat and cholesterol, may reduce the risk of heart disease." Some studies that proved the benefits of beta glucan used pretty large amounts of the fiber, but a review of the research found adding as little as 10 g of fiber per day to your menu could reduce your LDL by an average of 22 points. A hearty breakfast is a good start, since you can get that much fiber in two and a half cups of cooked oatmeal. Eating oatmeal is one easy thing you can do every day to flush out your arteries and lower your cholesterol.

Beta glucan is a health winner in other ways. It helps speed waste products through your digestive system before they can do damage, thus lowering your risk of colon cancer. It may also help keep your blood pressure down.

Get a grip on diabetes. People with diabetes know they should add more fiber to their diets. That could include both insoluble fiber, the kind that doesn't break down or get absorbed from the food you eat, and soluble fiber, the kind that forms a gooey gel in your intestines. Research has shown that a high-fiber diet may lower blood levels of insulin and glucose — sugar in your blood. Oatmeal is a great choice for controlling diabetes because of its soluble fiber, beta glucan. It moves slowly through your intestines, taking longer to digest. That means your blood sugar doesn't rise so quickly after a meal. And because fiber fills you up, it inhibits weight gain as well.

Eating more fiber may even help you avoid type 2 diabetes in the first place. Fiber helps because it slows down the digestion of carbohydrates into glucose. That means your body will pump out less insulin than it would if you ate food with little fiber. Researchers tested this idea among a group of 36,000 older women in Iowa. Those who ate at least 7.5 grams (g) of cereal fiber every day were 36 percent less likely to develop diabetes than the women who ate less than half as much. And 7.5 g is not a lot of fiber. You can get 4 g of fiber in a single bowl of oatmeal.

■ ■ ■ ■ ■ Boost the benefits ■ ■ ■ ■ ■

Picking the best choice for breakfast or baking can bewilder even the most devoted oatmeal lover. Some types cook quickly, while others provide greater nutritional benefits. Here is a list of key oatmeal players from the least to the most processed.

- Oat groats. These hulled and roasted whole oats cook in 30 to 40 minutes.

- Steel-cut oats. Also known as Scottish or Irish oats, these whole oats have been roasted and cut into small pieces. They cook in about 15 minutes.

- Old-fashioned rolled oats. Steaming and flattening oat kernels further reduces cooking time.

- Quick-cooking oats. These flattened oats are cut even more finely for quicker cooking.

- Instant oatmeal. You can prepare this dish by adding boiling water because the oats are rolled thin and pre-cooked. But because some flavor may be lost during the process, they often have added sugar and salt.

Prostate protection is easy to come by. There is good news about prostate cancer — you can take charge of your risk through what you eat. Oatmeal is one very smart choice.

Again, it's a whole grain with a high fiber content. Experts believe a diet with lots of fiber — not the typical Western diet — may help because of how fiber works with sex hormones. Fiber latches on to sex steroids, then when the fiber leaves your body, out go the excess hormones, too. Because male hormones are linked to growth of prostate tumors, that's a good thing.

The other benefit of oatmeal is that it's high in selenium, a trace mineral that acts as an antioxidant. It works with vitamin E to help your immune system function and lower your testosterone level. One study of older men in Baltimore found that those with less selenium in their blood were more likely to develop prostate cancer. An ongoing long-term study may give a stronger answer about selenium's power against the disease. Results of the Selenium and Vitamin E Cancer Prevention Trial (SELECT) will be available in 2013.

As with many vitamins and minerals, you don't want to overdo selenium. Too much can cause belly pain, arthritis, emotional problems, hair loss, and liver problems. In fact, some experts say only men who don't get enough selenium can benefit from increasing the mineral in their diets. A bowl of oatmeal every morning is a simple way to get about 19 micrograms, or 27 percent of your daily requirement.

Gluten free? Skip the oatmeal

Oatmeal may not be such a comforting food if you have celiac disease. People with this condition have an immune reaction to the gluten in wheat, barley, rye, and other grains. Gluten flattens out the villi, or fingerlike projections, in their intestines so nutrients can't be absorbed as well. This can lead to malnutrition, diarrhea, bloating, and other troubles. Avoiding gluten usually solves the problem.

New research shows pure oats don't have gluten, but it typically gets into the grain during processing. You may need to stay away from oatmeal — and everything made from oats — if you're on a gluten-free diet.

Enjoy a skin-soothing tubful of comfort. A hearty bowl of oatmeal is comforting for your innards, and a tubful of the stuff works wonders on your skin. You can buy oatmeal-containing lotions that claim to soothe dry, irritated skin. Turns out this promise is not all fluff. Colloidal oatmeal, or the finely ground powdery form, can protect your skin and fight itching and irritation from poison ivy, insect bites, chickenpox, and other causes. It acts as a barrier to hold in moisture and relieve dry skin — along with the irritation that comes with it.

Put this remedy to work by mixing up your own bath of colloidal oatmeal and soaking for a spell. You can put regular oatmeal in a food processor and grind it up, then add about two cups to your bath. Be careful as you step into the tub, since it will be slippery.

▪ ▪ ▪ ▪ *Cook's corner* ▪ ▪ ▪ ▪

Price and nutritional content vary depending on the form of your oatmeal. You pay more — in dollars and in nutrition — for convenience. Check out these comparisons before you buy.

Type of oatmeal	Price per serving	Calories per serving	Fiber (grams per serving)	Sugar (grams per serving)
Regular oatmeal (plain)	$0.20	147	4	1
Quaker Instant (baked apple)	$0.44	153	3	14
Quaker Oatmeal Express (baked apple)	$1.39	208	4	19
Quaker Oatmeal To Go (bar, baked apple)	$0.55	220	5	21

New food labels simplify going gluten-free

Taking certain foods out of your diet can be tricky. That's doubly true with an ingredient like gluten, a protein in wheat and other grains that causes trouble for people with celiac disease. Gluten can hide in places you don't expect, like lipstick, postage stamps, medicines, or foods like processed meats, imitation bacon, and sauces. But new rules should make it easier to avoid gluten.

The U.S. Food and Drug Administration (FDA) is proposing new rules for foods that claim to be "gluten-free" on the label. Companies could call foods "gluten-free" if they don't have wheat, barley, rye, or related grains like spelt and triticale — and don't have more than 20 parts per million (ppm) of gluten. The new rules also say foods that don't usually have gluten, like meat or milk, can call themselves "gluten-free" if they include a phrase like "all milk is gluten-free." An exception is oats, which don't have gluten in their natural form but can easily be contaminated as they're processed. For that reason, experts recommend celiac sufferers avoid oat products as well.

What's so bad about gluten? Some people blame sensitivity to gluten for symptoms of autism in children, along with fatigue, joint pain, excess weight, yeast infections, and other illnesses in adults. Experts don't all blame gluten for these problems, but they agree it's off limits for people with celiac disease, also called sprue. In these folks, gluten harms villi in the small intestines so they can't absorb nutrients well. This causes weight loss, anemia, bloating, and diarrhea, and it can lead to osteoporosis.

People sensitive to gluten want to know if foods have even a small amount, but the FDA has settled on a 20-ppm limit. They say such a low level shouldn't cause problems, and most tests are reliable for that small amount.

Quinoa

■ ■ ■ ■ ■ ■ ■ ■ ■ ■ ■

'Super grain' packs a nutritional punch

The Incas called it the "mother seed" because it was so important, and its name came from the Spanish word for "fantastic." A wonderful taste earns it the nickname "vegetarian caviar," and wonderful nutrition means it's been called the "super grain of the future." Since it was brought to the United States and planted in the 1980s, quinoa (pronounced "keen-wah") has lived up to its reputation for goodness, even if it's not yet well known.

Like amaranth, quinoa is not really a grain. It's a grass plant with edible seeds and leaves you can serve like spinach. Most people who eat quinoa cook the seeds like rice or hot cereal, or they use the flour to make pancakes, cookies, or muffins.

Quinoa is a whole grain with lots of fiber; minerals like iron, copper, manganese, magnesium, and phosphorus; and B vitamins such as thiamin, niacin, and riboflavin. It's full of energy, and it can fill you up better than traditional grains like wheat. But don't think of quinoa as a diet food. One cup of quinoa has 636 calories — nearly three times as many as brown rice.

Surefire cure for anemia. Do you feel weak and tired a lot? Have trouble fighting off sickness? Feel cold or hot when nobody around you does? You may not be getting enough iron

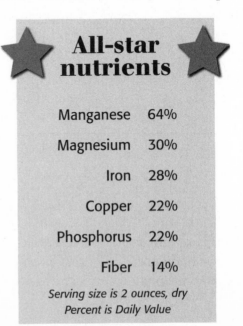

All-star nutrients

Manganese	64%
Magnesium	30%
Iron	28%
Copper	22%
Phosphorus	22%
Fiber	14%

Serving size is 2 ounces, dry
Percent is Daily Value

234

in your diet. You need iron, an essential mineral, so red blood cells can carry oxygen to your body. That's why not getting enough iron can make you tired and weak. You may feel the effects of too little iron even if you don't technically have anemia.

Popeye the sailor knew how important iron was for his health and strength — "I fights to the finish, 'cause I eats my spinach." But in reality, quinoa is a better source of iron than spinach is. A 2-ounce serving of quinoa delivers 28 percent of the iron you'll need in a day. That's more than five times the iron you get from one cup of raw spinach.

Along with preventing iron-deficiency anemia, the right amount of iron may help you think more clearly, keep your bones strong after menopause, and stave off restless legs syndrome.

■ ■ ■ ■ ■ **Boost the benefits** ■ ■ ■ ■ ■

Most grains don't have a balanced blend of the amino acids your body needs. Not so with quinoa, which has 8 grams of protein in a 2-ounce serving. Even better, it's a balanced, high-quality protein that has lots of lysine — the essential amino acid other grains tend to lack. In fact, quinoa is such a good source of protein the United Nations Food and Agricultural Organization puts it in the same category as dried whole milk. Another benefit is that people who can't eat gluten can enjoy quinoa since it's gluten free.

Copper helps banish bone loss. Quinoa is a great source of other important minerals, including magnesium, manganese, phosphorus, and copper. Yes, that's right — that same shiny metal used in cookware and jewelry is also great for your health. Copper helps your body use iron to make red blood cells, and it works with calcium to keep your bones strong as you age.

Copper is part of an enzyme, lysyl oxidase, that helps your body make collagen, the fiber that gives structure to strong bones. Experts think it may play a role in helping prevent osteoporosis, the bone loss that often happens as you age. Osteoporosis can lead to fractures and a stooped-over posture because of small breaks in your spine. But studies show women during and after menopause who took copper supplements for two years had less bone loss than those who skipped the copper.

A 2-ounce serving of quinoa provides 22 percent of the copper you need, so start your day with a hearty bowl of good bone health. You can pour on some calcium-rich milk for even better osteoporosis protection.

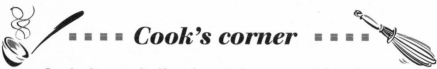

▪ ▪ ▪ ▪ *Cook's corner* ▪ ▪ ▪ ▪

Soak the seeds. If you've tried quinoa and found it bitter tasting, maybe you didn't soak it long enough. The seeds naturally have a soapy coating called saponin to keep away birds and insects. Wash it off before you cook quinoa. Seeds you buy are usually pre-washed, but a bit more rinsing won't hurt. There is so much saponin on the seeds that some native people in Bolivia use the rinse water as a shampoo.

Cook it quickly. Quinoa seeds cook in about 15 minutes— twice as fast as rice. Boil them using about two cups of liquid for each cup of seeds.

Make your own flour. You can make quinoa flour by grinding the seeds in a blender or nut grinder. Store the flour in the refrigerator to keep it from turning rancid.

Try it in all its variety. If you don't like the idea of cooking up a bowl of quinoa seeds, you can buy it as cereal flakes, in snack bars, or added to dried pasta.

4 secrets to healthy pasta sauce

You made the switch from regular pasta to whole-wheat noodles. That's great — you're getting B vitamins, fiber, and about 200 calories in a 2-ounce serving. Pasta is an inexpensive meal that's filling and tasty. But don't sabotage your good-health efforts by choosing the wrong pasta sauce. Keep these ideas in mind when you select a sauce.

- Pick red over white. Sauces that are white, like alfredo sauce, typically have more fat and calories — from cheese and cream — than red sauces like marinara. And redder tomato sauces give you more of the cancer-fighting nutrient lycopene.

- Get saucy with veggies. Punch up the nutrient content of sauce in a jar by adding your own chopped vegetables. Try broccoli, carrots, or red peppers.

- Check the label. Pasta sauce in a jar is convenient, but notice what might be added. Some contain loads of sugar and salt.

- Watch your portions. Your pasta doesn't need to go for a swim in its sauce. A reasonable amount of marinara sauce is a half cup, while specialty sauces like pesto are usually served by the quarter cup.

These popular pasta sauces all taste great — but see how ingredients make a great nutritional difference.

Sauce (1/2 cup)	Calories	Fat (g)	Sodium (mg)
Classico Tomato & Basil	60	1	310
Prego Hearty Meat Three-Meat Supreme	170	10	600
Ragu Classic Alfredo	220	20	800
Classico Traditional Basil Pesto (1/4 cup)	230	21	720

Spelt

■ ■ ■ ■ ■ ■ ■ ■

Wheat substitute boasts all-around benefits

If there were a "saint of spelt," her name would be Hildegard. A nun from the twelfth century, Hildegard of Bingen believed in the healing powers of the grain, a close cousin to wheat. She wrote that eating spelt, "the very best grain," would make you healthier, stronger, and more beautiful. Spelt was popular in Europe for centuries before wheat — with its easily removed husks and greater yields — became the rage.

Hildegard may have been on the right track when she urged sick people to eat the easily digestible spelt. Some people with allergies to wheat can eat spelt, so it makes a good substitute in baked items. On the other hand, spelt has gluten, the protein that people with celiac disease are avoiding when they shun wheat products. If you are sensitive to wheat, talk to your doctor to see if spelt can grace your plate.

But spelt is jam-packed with nutrients that can help your body in other ways. Compared to wheat, spelt has fewer calories and more B vitamins and minerals like manganese, copper, iron, potassium, and zinc. Spelt lovers appreciate how easily this fibrous food is digested — the grains practically melt in your mouth — and how good it tastes. You and your body will love it.

Natural remedy for migraine pain. If you're among the many people who suffer from throbbing pain on one side of your

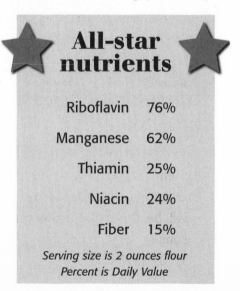

All-star nutrients

Riboflavin	76%
Manganese	62%
Thiamin	25%
Niacin	24%
Fiber	15%

Serving size is 2 ounces flour
Percent is Daily Value

head, nausea, and light sensitivity, you'd like some relief. The answer may be spelled "spelt."

Studies show taking a large dose of riboflavin, or vitamin B2, may prevent migraines. In one four-month study, people who took 400 milligrams (mg) of a riboflavin supplement daily had 50 percent fewer migraine attacks. That means half as many days of lost work, golfing, gardening, or playing with your grandchildren.

Experts think riboflavin helps cells use energy better to prevent migraines. Riboflavin is a water-soluble vitamin, and you can get it in foods like fortified cereals, dairy products, eggs — and spelt. But a quarter of seniors don't get enough. You'd have to eat a lot of spelt to get 400 mg, but you may not be able to absorb more than 25 mg at once anyway. You can get a good start if you substitute spelt for wheat. Just 2 ounces of spelt flour has 1.3 mg, or 76 percent of the riboflavin you should get every day. Some people think the visions of Saint Hildegard of Bingen were caused by migraines. If it's true, maybe that's another reason she was so fond of spelt.

■ ■ ■ ■ ■ Boost the benefits ■ ■ ■ ■ ■

Don't waste space on your plate for foods that have little good-health value. Cook up a spelt side dish that beats out white rice when it comes to nutrition. An equal serving of spelt has fewer calories yet more protein, phosphorous, potassium, and riboflavin than white rice. Spelt also boasts less sodium and a dozen times more fiber than white rice.

Soak spelt berries (whole kernels) overnight, then drain them and put in water to boil for 45 to 60 minutes. Use 3 cups of water for each 1 1/4 cup of spelt. They will be chewy but tender and ready for your favorite seasonings. One cup of raw spelt more than doubles when it's cooked.

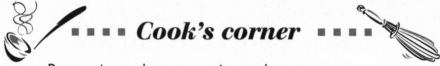

Cook's corner

Be creative, and you can enjoy spelt at every meal. Look for these items in a grocery or health-food store.

- Flaked spelt is made into a dry breakfast cereal similar to corn or bran flakes. You can also add spelt berries or flakes to granola or cook them like oatmeal.

- Spelt pastas let you enjoy your favorite Italian dishes with this high-protein grain. Try spaghetti, penne, macaroni elbows, lasagna, and more.

- Snack on spelt in the form of crackers, flat bread, puffed cakes similar to rice cakes, and pretzels. You'll find flavors like garlic, cheddar, or sour cream and onion — like potato chips, only healthier.

- Spelt flour works in many recipes that call for wheat flour, so you can make bread, cookies, cakes — whatever you like. Because spelt flour has more moisture than wheat flour, you'll probably need to add less liquid when you bake with it. Experiment to get the taste just right.

- Pay attention to whether you're buying whole-grain or refined spelt flour. Just as with wheat, refining spelt grains removes the bran, germ, and lots of nutrition.

Basic rules for buying healthier breads

Even if you mean to buy whole grains, you may be stumped by the words used on bread packages. Here are some basic rules to be sure your breads — or flour tortillas, pita bread, or buns — are truly whole grain, which means they're made from the entire grain of wheat.

- Bread made from only whole grains should say "100-percent whole grains" on the label. Phrases like "wheat bread," "stone ground," "multigrain," or "made from whole wheat" do not show the bread is whole grain.

- Bread's color doesn't prove its health value. Some brown breads get their color from molasses or caramel food coloring — not from whole grains.

- The U.S. Food and Drug Administration lets companies include this language on products that contain 51 percent or more whole-grain ingredients by weight: "Diets rich in whole grain foods and other plant foods, and low in total fat, saturated fat, and cholesterol, may reduce the risk of heart disease and certain cancers."

- If you love pumpernickel, you should know it's often not whole grain. The bread is made from rye and wheat flours. Similarly, most U.S. rye bread is not whole grain.

People hooked on white bread may like new "Ultragrain" bread, or whole-grain bread that appears white. It's made from white hard wheat instead of the traditional red wheat. That makes the flour lighter and sweeter — more like white bread. The only problem is bread manufacturers are not yet using 100-percent Ultragrain flour but blending it with refined flour.

Wheat bran

Tap the power of the outer grain

Take a grain of wheat and scrape away the bran and germ, and you're left with the starchy center — and not much nutrition. That's how wheat is milled to make white bread, and that's why it must be enriched to add back the missing vitamins and minerals. Most of the grain's vitamins, minerals, protein, and fiber are in the wheat bran. That's what makes wheat bran, the outer coating of the grain, such a great addition to breakfast cereals and muffins.

You might hear bread called the "staff of life," but the term really fits wheat bran. This outer part of the whole-wheat grain is known for having lots of insoluble fiber. It's also a great source of some B vitamins like niacin, along with important minerals like magnesium, selenium, and phosphorous. Wheat bran offers loads of the essential mineral manganese, which your body uses to make enzymes, shore up your immune system, and build strong bones.

Of course, you can get lots of wheat bran in some tasty breakfast cereals, like All-Bran and Raisin Bran. But you can also add wheat bran to your favorite bread and muffin recipes, or you can try all kinds of recipes that include wheat bran or bran cereals. Check out *www.all-bran.com* for ideas on adding wheat bran at breakfast, lunch, and dinner. And don't forget the simplest way to add

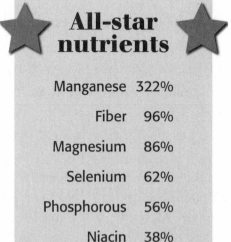

All-star nutrients

Manganese	322%
Fiber	96%
Magnesium	86%
Selenium	62%
Phosphorous	56%
Niacin	38%

Serving size is 2 ounces, dry
Percent is Daily Value

wheat bran to your diet: switch from white bread to 100 percent whole-wheat bread.

Dodge colon cancer and digestive woes. You may have heard that eating more fiber may help prevent cancer of the colon, or large intestine. Experts are debating whether this is true or whether it's the other nutrients in plant foods that protect your colon. It's also possible that people who eat lots of fiber-filled plant foods simply eat less meat, which has been found to raise your risk. But there are a couple of great reasons why whole-grain foods may be your colon's best friend.

- Phytic acid, a natural chemical found in wheat bran and other plants, works like an antioxidant to stop tumor growth.

- Wheat bran has oodles of insoluble fiber. With 24 grams of fiber in a 2-ounce serving, wheat bran gives you nearly a full day's worth of fiber. That fiber adds bulk to stool in your intestines, moving carcinogens along and out of your body quickly — before they get a chance to cause trouble. All that fiber also may help prevent constipation.

The fiber in wheat bran helps other parts of your body as well. Eating it every day may help beat fatigue and give you a more positive attitude. Adding insoluble fiber to your diet is also one way to fool your body into keeping your weight in check. An eight-year study of middle-aged men found those who ate more whole-grain foods gained less weight. For every 20 grams per day more fiber they ate, men gained 12 pounds less during the study. Experts say insoluble fiber — like the kind in wheat bran — helps fill you up faster so you eat less. Whole-grain foods have lots of fiber and water so they contain fewer calories than similar refined grains. Do your digestion a favor and eat a fiber-filled cereal daily.

Give gum disease the heave-ho. Along with their other benefits, whole-grain breads and cereals may help protect you from gingivitis, also known as gum disease. Sound too good to be true? Not so. Researchers tested this idea by studying 34,000 middle-aged men for 14 years. Men who ate about three and a half servings of whole grains every day had healthier gums. In fact, they were 23 percent less likely to have gum disease than the men who ate less than one serving a day.

The researchers think eating more whole grains lets your body absorb carbohydrates more slowly in the intestines. That means blood sugar levels stay constant and your body suffers less inflammation. It all leads to healthier gums in the long run.

■ ■ ■ ■ ■ **Boost the benefits** ■ ■ ■ ■ ■

Bake whole-wheat pizza crust longer and at a higher temperature, and you may be cooking up better health. That's what researchers discovered when they looked for ways to make pizza healthier. They found cooking whole-wheat pizza crust at 550 degrees Fahrenheit and for about 14 minutes, rather than seven, caused more antioxidants to be released from the wheat bran. Antioxidants are natural chemicals that help your cells repair damage to avoid all kinds of illnesses. The scientists also suggest letting pizza dough ferment for a long period of time, up to 48 hours, for a bigger antioxidant boost.

Do double duty for your heart. Many studies show eating whole grains instead of refined grains may help protect you from heart disease and heart failure. You probably know oatmeal, with its soluble fiber, can lower your cholesterol. But how can wheat bran help your heart?

■ Trade in your bacon-and-eggs breakfast for whole-grain cereal, and you'll cut your risk of heart disease. Besides skipping a couple servings of saturated fats and cholesterol, you're adding insoluble fiber to your diet. One study found people who ate the most whole grains had the least risk of heart disease and diabetes. Researchers suggest the fiber in whole-grain foods keeps blood sugar from rising as quickly, and they think the other nutrients in whole grain also help protect your heart.

- Wheat bran is high in magnesium, an essential mineral that helps keep your heart rhythm steady and your blood pressure stable. It's sometimes called "nature's calcium channel blocker" because it works like some heart drugs to relax blood vessels and treat high blood pressure. In one study, men who got more magnesium in their diets — along with potassium and fiber — had less chance of high blood pressure.

Two ounces of wheat bran give you nearly all the fiber and magnesium you need in a day. Make it part of your personal heart-smart diet.

▪ ▪ ▪ ▪ *Cook's corner* ▪ ▪ ▪ ▪

If you're in the habit of buying whichever wheat flour is on sale, think again. Various types behave differently in cooking and baking — to say nothing of their nutritional content. Here is a rundown of some common types of flour.

- **All-purpose or enriched flour.** This processed white flour has no wheat bran or wheat germ, making it less nutritious than whole-wheat flour. It's used for general cooking or baking.

- **Self-rising flour.** Made from all-purpose flour, this variety has added salt, leavening like baking powder or soda, and an acid-releasing ingredient. The leavening begins to lose its power in two months, so use it fast or throw it out.

- **Unbleached wheat flour.** This is simply all-purpose flour that hasn't been bleached. It may have some of the wheat bran and germ added back.

- Bread flour. About 98 percent of this product is high-gluten hard wheat flour. Malted barley is added to improve yeast activity.

- Graham flour. Developed in the 19th century as an alternative to white flour, this coarse brown whole-wheat flour makes tasty but dense bread.

- WheatSelect flour. This newly developed flour from Horizon Mills looks and feels a lot like white flour, but it has most of the good nutrition of whole wheat.

Beef up your protein with beans and legumes

Black beans

■ ■ ■ ■ ■ ■ ■ ■ ■ ■ ■ ■ ■ ■ ■ ■ ■ ■

Cheap staple helps thwart disease

Mexican food just wouldn't be the same without this longtime staple. Black beans have carved out a prime place on people's plates in refried beans, burritos, black bean soup, and cold bean salads.

Experts think common beans originated in Central America, where archeologists have found the remains of 7,000 year-old beans. Columbus and the Spanish and Portuguese explorers who came after him took these beans back to Europe and on to Asia.

Now they're everywhere, and for good reason. There are as many different kinds of beans as there are health benefits, but this is one 50-cent meal that can keep your arteries clear. Also known as turtle beans, black beans are fairly bursting with healthy benefits, like high-quality protein, B vitamins, and minerals. Plus, as a legume, they're one of the best food sources of soluble fiber. All this adds up to lower cholesterol and fewer problems with heart disease, diabetes, and many other serious conditions.

Put a halt to heart problems. According to the American Heart Association, more than 79 million Americans suffer from high blood pressure, heart attack, angina, stroke, or a combination of these illnesses — all different forms of cardiovascular disease (CVD). But eating black beans and other folate-filled legumes regularly could drop-kick your CVD risk as much as 90 percent.

The B vitamin folate helps your body process a protein

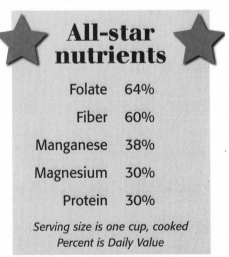

All-star nutrients

Folate	64%
Fiber	60%
Manganese	38%
Magnesium	30%
Protein	30%

Serving size is one cup, cooked
Percent is Daily Value

called homocysteine and keep it from building up in your blood. In normal amounts, homocysteine is harmless. But in large amounts, it can lead to narrowing and plaque buildup in your arteries.

■ ■ ■ ■ ■ Boost the benefits ■ ■ ■ ■ ■

Refried beans may taste great, but all that processing puts sugar into your bloodstream faster, leading to after-meal spikes in blood sugar and insulin — a particular danger if you have diabetes or prediabetes.

You're better off eating whole beans because you digest their starches more slowly. In fact, your body may not completely digest unprocessed legumes, so some sugars may never even make it to your bloodstream. Plus, unrefined beans make you feel full longer, which can help with weight loss.

More than 80 studies suggest even moderately high levels of homocysteine in your blood increases your risk for developing CVD. That's where high-folate foods like black beans come in. A Finnish study on nearly 2,000 men found those who ate the most folate-rich foods had a 55 percent lower risk of a serious heart event, like a heart attack, compared to those who ate the least.

In a recent analysis of 25 high-quality studies, researchers concluded that getting as little as 200 micrograms (mcg) of folate daily could lower homocysteine levels 60 percent. Getting 400 mcg drops it a whopping 90 percent, which makes black beans the way to go. Just a cup of these humble legumes gives you 256 mcg of folate.

While studies have proven that higher homocysteine raises your risk for CVD, none have proven that lowering homocysteine reduces your risk. Still, eating a balanced diet with plenty of folate and other B vitamins can't hurt.

Folate isn't the only vitamin you need to fight high homocysteine and CVD risk. Vitamins B6 and B12 are also involved in processing this protein. Too little of them can also lead to high homocysteine. For the biggest benefit, experts say you need to eat foods like spinach, bananas, and potatoes for plenty of B6, plus low-fat milk, lean beef, and shellfish for B12.

Control the ups and downs of diabetes. Black beans pack a three-part punch for preventing type 2 diabetes plus helping you manage blood sugar and insulin levels if you already have it.

■ *Magnesium.* Experts think low levels of this mineral contribute to the development of type 2 diabetes. Once you have it, diabetes itself makes you lose more magnesium through your urine. It's a vicious cycle but one you can help break by eating more magnesium-rich foods like black beans. A review of eight studies showed people who got the most magnesium in their diet had a 23 percent lower risk of type 2 diabetes. Other research suggests boosting low magnesium levels may improve glucose tolerance in older adults and people who already have diabetes.

■ *Soluble fiber.* The major fiber found in beans, barley, and oats slows down your absorption of sugar from food. This helps control spikes in blood sugar and insulin after meals, an important goal in fighting diabetes. Experts say you need to eat at least 5 to 6 grams (g) of soluble fiber each day to get these benefits. Black beans top the legume list in soluble fiber, with a whopping 4.8 g per cooked cup.

■ *Resistant starch.* You may not think of starches as good for diabetes, but they are if you eat the right kind. Some foods, like beans and bananas, contain resistant starches (RS), a special type of insoluble fiber that makes your stubborn cells more sensitive to insulin. Scientists say you need to eat a minimum of 5 to 6 g of RS daily to boost your insulin sensitivity. Most cooked beans pack between 1 and 1.75 grams of RS per cup.

Eating meals that combine foods high in RS with those rich in soluble fiber appear to control insulin and balance blood sugar better than either nutrient alone. Beans boast both, making them a good choice for diabetes control.

Block bone loss with important mineral. Women with osteoporosis may have lower levels of the mineral manganese than women with healthy bones. Once again, black beans come to the rescue as a naturally good source of this essential mineral. A few studies suggest that getting more manganese may slow or even prevent bone loss in postmenopausal women. That makes sense since your body needs it to form bones and cartilage. Antacids and laxatives made with magnesium keep your body from absorbing manganese efficiently, so avoid taking them alongside a manganese-rich meal.

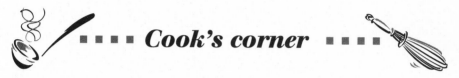

Cook's corner

Uncooked, dried beans will keep up to a year in a sealed container in a cool, dark place. You can also freeze dried beans indefinitely. Cooked beans can last up to five days in the refrigerator.

You don't have to skip beans to avoid gas. Try these tips to cut down on this unsociable side effect and still reap the benefits of good nutrition.

- Change the water at least twice during soaking and again during cooking.

- Add a few drops of an anti-gas product like Beano to beans before serving them. It packs an enzyme that breaks down the complex sugars that cause gas before they get in your stomach.

- Add beans to your diet gradually, but eat them often. Beans will cause less gas if you eat them regularly.

Chickpeas

■ ■ ■ ■ ■ ■ ■ ■ ■ ■ ■ ■ ■ ■ ■ ■

Nutty beans deliver big benefits

Garbanzo beans, otherwise known as chickpeas, are one of the most versatile and flavorful legumes. Humans began eating these beans roughly 7,000 years ago. Ancient Egyptians, Hebrews, Greeks, and Romans have all enjoyed their nutty taste.

No wonder. Chickpeas are chock full of fiber and healthy polyunsaturated fats (PUFAs), and a gold mine of copper, manganese, and folate. Plus, they boast special phytochemicals known as isoflavones, the same ones that make soybeans so famous.

Any way you can imagine, you can probably eat chickpeas. Serve them hot as a side dish or cold sprinkled over salad. Stir them into a hearty minestrone soup in true Italian style, or mash them to make a yummy hummus dip. You can even buy them roasted and salted, just like peanuts. Need more convincing? Check out the following ways they improve your health.

Put the brakes on cancer. Nitrosamines are cancer-causing compounds that you encounter almost every day. They show up in everything from meat and milk products to soft drinks, tobacco, and alcohol. When they enter your digestive tract, they raise your risk of stomach, bladder, and esophageal cancer. When you get them from smoking or chewing tobacco, they contribute to the development of lung, mouth, and throat cancers.

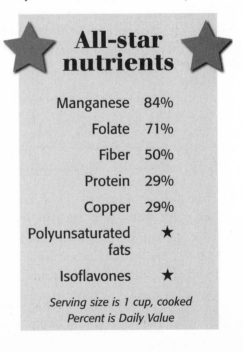

All-star nutrients

Manganese	84%
Folate	71%
Fiber	50%
Protein	29%
Copper	29%
Polyunsaturated fats	★
Isoflavones	★

Serving size is 1 cup, cooked
Percent is Daily Value

■ ■ ■ ■ ■ **Boost the benefits** ■ ■ ■ ■ ■

Like most legumes, chickpeas pack a lot of protein, but it's incomplete. Protein from these beans lacks the amino acids methionine and cystine. However, it does contain lots of lysine. Try combining your chickpeas with grains, which offer plenty of methionine and cystine but no lysine. Together, each makes up for what the other lacks, so eating a meal that includes both chickpeas and grains will give you complete protein.

A delicious hummus dip is one way to strike this balance. This Middle Eastern favorite combines puréed chickpeas, good-for-you garlic, olive oil, lemon juice, paprika, and other flavorful spices. Dip in your favorite whole-grain bread for a protein-packed appetizer any guest will enjoy.

Once inside your body, these dangerous compounds wreak havoc by churning out free radicals that damage your cells and trigger disease-causing changes. But researchers say the fiber in chickpeas may protect you by keeping your body from absorbing nitrosamines. The fewer you absorb, the less damage they do.

This doesn't mean eating chickpeas will prevent lung cancer if you smoke or will offset other bad habits. You still need to take care of your body. However, making these beans a regular part of your diet could give you another layer of protection against diseases and aging, while adding variety to your meals.

Lose the fat and lower cholesterol. Of all the legumes, chickpeas may be the best at cutting your cholesterol. Experts chalk it up to three big benefits of these beans — fiber, polyunsaturated fats (PUFAs), and isoflavones. These nutrients seem to work together to control cholesterol, trim body fat, and improve insulin sensitivity.

In an Australian study, people who ate a regular diet supplemented with canned chickpeas and chickpea flour lowered their total and LDL cholesterol levels, compared to people who got most of their fiber from wheat and cereal. In all, these bean-eaters got 27 grams of fiber — about two cups of chickpeas — daily. What's more, their change in cholesterol earned them a 13.5 percent drop in heart disease risk.

A Chinese study had similar results. Normally, rats fed a high-fat diet become obese and insulin resistant, and develop high cholesterol. But when these rats got chickpeas in addition to all that fat, they actually lost belly fat, lowered their LDL cholesterol, and improved their ratio of HDL to LDL.

Chickpeas are good news for people at risk for type 2 diabetes, too. The amount of body fat you carry largely determines how resistant your cells are to insulin. Insulin resistance, in turn, is a precursor to full-blown, type 2 diabetes. Sure enough, when these obese rats lost their extra fat on the chickpea diet, they also reversed their insulin resistance.

■ ■ ■ ■ *Cook's corner* ■ ■ ■ ■

Dried chickpeas are harder than most other beans, so they need to soak a bit longer. Soak them for 12 to 16 hours overnight, then boil for two to two and half hours or until tender. You can shorten the cooking time in two ways.

■ In a pressure cooker, cook soaked beans 20 to 25 minutes or unsoaked beans 35 to 40 minutes. Add a tablespoon of oil to prevent foaming, which may clog the vent.

■ Prepare dried beans now for quick cooking later by soaking them overnight, then freezing them in the same water. When you're ready to eat them, simply thaw beforehand and cook for one hour less than normal.

Lentils

■ ■ ■ ■ ■ ■ ■ ■ ■ ■

Ancient legume offers timely healing

Lentils have been a hot property for more than 8,000 years. In fact, they are one of the oldest cultivated crops in the world. In the Bible, Esau sold his birthright as the eldest son to Jacob, his younger brother, just for a bowl of red lentils. Luckily, you don't have to pay that much.

Some of the healthiest foods are actually the cheapest — like lentils, a 50-cent meal that can help you lose weight and lower your cholesterol. They may even protect you from cancer, diabetes, and macular degeneration. Not bad for a humble food.

These legumes are also an inexpensive source of protein for people around the world. Half a cup of lentils gives you about the same protein as one ounce of lean, cooked meat. Plus, they're an excellent source of folate, phosphorous, fiber, and iron.

Easy way to banish flab for good. Lentils may be the perfect weight-loss food. They make you feel full longer and help you shed fat, while supplying important nutrients. High-protein foods like lentils trigger your body to release a hunger-squashing hormone known as PYY. The more PYY released, the fuller you feel and the less you eat. Lentils fit the bill as an excellent source of plant protein with very little saturated fat or cholesterol, unlike protein from most meat and dairy sources.

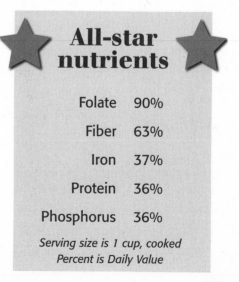

All-star nutrients

Folate	90%
Fiber	63%
Iron	37%
Protein	36%
Phosphorus	36%

Serving size is 1 cup, cooked
Percent is Daily Value

■ ■ ■ ■ ■ **Boost the benefits** ■ ■ ■ ■ ■

Lentils are a good source of phosphorous but not calcium. To keep these two minerals in balance, be sure to eat high-calcium, low-phosphorous foods such as turnip greens or TOTAL corn flakes cereal on days you serve up lentils.

Like most other legumes, lentils contain protein that lacks the amino acids methionine and lysine. Eat them in a meal with grains to balance out the missing amino acids, and you'll end up with complete protein.

To make them easier for sensitive digestive systems to digest, simply plunge washed lentils directly into boiling water.

Lentils are also a low-GI food, and new research shows eating a low-GI diet helps you lose more weight than other diets. The GI, or Glycemic Index, is a measure of how quickly the carbohydrates in a food turn into sugar and enter your bloodstream. The longer they take, the lower the food's GI rating.

An important review of six studies found low-GI diets do, indeed, help people lose weight, especially obese people. Those eating low-GI foods lost more body fat and more weight than people on other weight-loss diets in one recent study. The GI-watchers also slashed their total cholesterol and LDL cholesterol levels — important risk factors for heart problems. The best part — they could eat as much as they wanted, as long as they ate mostly low-GI foods like lentils. In fact, the more they ate, the more weight they lost. Other research finds that people who eat mostly low-GI foods, like lentils, typically weigh less than people eating mostly high-GI foods, like white bread.

Serving up lentils in soup can help you drop even more pounds. Broth-based soups with healthy ingredients like legumes have few calories but take up lots of space in your stomach, so you feel full. Snack bars and crackers with the same number of calories take up much less space, leaving you still hungry. The results of one weight-loss study prove this point — substituting a low-calorie soup for a dry snack twice a day can help you lose 50 percent more weight than dieting alone. And on a diet like that, you won't feel starved.

Arm your eyes against AMD. Lentils' low GI-value may benefit your eyes as well. In a study of more than 500 women spanning 10 years, those who ate the most high-GI foods were more than twice as likely to develop early age-related macular degeneration (AMD).

Chronically high blood sugar, caused by eating high-GI foods, may lead to inflammation and oxidative damage in the delicate tissues of your eye. What's more, this study suggests even moderately high sugar levels, not high enough to qualify as diabetes, can damage your eyes.

Since nothing so far can cure AMD, experts say prevention is key. Make sure you eat mostly low-GI foods like lentils, vegetables, and whole grains, and keep high-GI foods, such as white bread and French fries, to a minimum. For the lowest GI, eat lentils whole, not mashed, and don't overcook them.

Cook up cancer-fighting power. Smoking and drinking are two habits that contribute to the development of cancer. Now add a folate-deficient diet to the list. Scientists say failing to get enough of this B vitamin is a long-term risk factor for certain cancers.

Folate is crucial in repairing DNA, the genetic material inside your cells. A shortage impairs your body's ability to repair damaged DNA, which in turn can lead to cancerous changes inside cells. Luckily, just one cup of lentils meets 90 percent of your folate needs for the day.

- Making high-folate foods part of your lifelong eating habits may protect you from cancer of the larynx. Italian researchers spent six months studying the effect of folic acid supplements in people with precancerous lesions. They found that almost half the people experienced a halt to their cancer while more than a fourth saw their lesions disappear.

- A study of Swedish men and women revealed that folate from foods, but not supplements, lowered the risk of pancreatic cancer. People who ate the most folate-rich foods were 25 percent less likely to develop the disease than those who ate the least. Taking folic acid supplements gave no protection. In fact, evidence suggests supplements may actually speed up the progression of pancreatic cancer in people who already have it.

Lentils pack more cancer-fighters than folate, though. The fiber and phytochemicals in lentils and other legumes could slash your colon cancer risk. Black men and women who ate dried beans, split peas, or lentils were nearly 20 percent less likely to develop colon cancer. A separate study linked eating lentils or beans twice a week to a 24 percent drop in breast cancer among women. In this case, researchers think phytochemicals called flavonols in legumes may hold the key. The moral of the story — you can't go wrong with lentils.

Enjoy double protection against diabetes. Foods that contain both soluble fiber and resistant starch, a special kind of starch that resists digestion, may protect against the development of type 2 diabetes and help people who have it better manage their blood sugar.

Fiber seems to slow the digestion of carbohydrates in a meal, so sugar hits your bloodstream more gradually instead of in a rush. Resistant starch may have similar effects, balancing after-meal blood sugar spikes, preventing bouts of low blood sugar, and lowering high blood sugar.

Research shows foods like lentils that boast both soluble fiber and resistant starch are best at controlling blood sugar and insulin levels. You need a minimum amount of fiber and resistant starch to gain these benefits, but you can reach those goals by eating at least one serving of lentils, barley flake cereal, an English muffin, and a citrus fruit every day.

▪ ▪ ▪ ▪ *Cook's corner* ▪ ▪ ▪ ▪

- Dried lentils are great time-savers because they cook quickly compared to other legumes. Rinse them first to wash off dust, dirt, and small stones. No need to soak them beforehand. Some varieties cook longer than others, so read the package directions. As with other beans, lengthen cooking time if you add acidic ingredients like tomatoes.

- These legumes come in a dizzying array of colors and uses. Substitute them for meat in meatloaf, or mix them with grains to bake breads and cakes. Look for lentil flour at the supermarket to make flat breads.

- Store uncooked lentils in an airtight container in a cool dry place up to a year. Or freeze them indefinitely.

Mung bean sprouts

Trim your waist, help your heart

The delicate, silvery shoots from sprouted mung beans are probably most familiar to you as an ingredient in chop suey. They are primarily grown in India and Pakistan and are a staple of Asian fare.

These nutty flavored shoots have lots of pros and few cons. They're mostly made up of water and other nutrients, which means they have very few calories or saturated fat. Plus, they're a good source of vitamin C, vitamin K, and phytosterols, heart-healthy compounds in plants. Start working these sprouts into sandwiches, soups, salads, and stir-fries for unique flavor and a bite of nutrition.

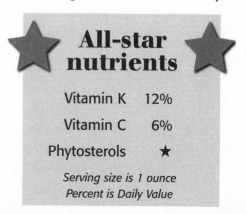

All-star nutrients

Vitamin K	12%
Vitamin C	6%
Phytosterols	★

Serving size is 1 ounce
Percent is Daily Value

▪ ▪ ▪ ▪ ▪ Boost the benefits ▪ ▪ ▪ ▪ ▪

To get the most out of your sprouts, eat them raw or stir-fried. Raw mung bean sprouts contain slightly more vitamins and minerals than boiled sprouts, and only raw sprouts have phytosterols. Stir-fried sprouts, on the other hand, contain no vitamin K but generally pack more vitamin C, B vitamins, and minerals than boiled or raw sprouts.

You can also buy bean sprouts canned and ready for serving, but they will be high in sodium. Rinse them first before adding them to your recipes.

Three keys to a hardier heart. Sprouts from mung beans supply three ingredients you need to guard your heart — vitamin K, vitamin C, and phytosterols.

- In cardiovascular disease, plaque builds up inside your arteries. Over time, these plaques harden and calcify, making your blood vessels less flexible and increasing your chance of blood clots, the main culprit behind heart attacks and strokes. Scientists aren't sure why, but having low levels of vitamin K in your blood makes these plaques more likely to calcify.

- Vitamin C relaxes blood vessels in people with angina, heart failure, high cholesterol and blood pressure, and clogged arteries. Clinical trials show vitamin C can also help lower blood pressure.

- Study after study has shown eating foods with phytosterols lowers both total and LDL cholesterol. These drops, in turn, can seriously cut your risk of heart disease.

Keep in mind, sprouts are tiny, and you generally eat them in small amounts. You'd need to eat a lot of mung bean sprouts to get substantial amounts of any nutrient. Think of them more as an added boost to a healthy diet, especially if you're trying to ward off heart woes.

Simple aid to weight loss. Mung bean sprouts are 90 percent water with fiber and nutrients thrown in for good measure. Adding them to sandwiches, stir-fried food, and soups gives you flavor and nutrition, but only a handful of calories. Bulking up your meals with foods that have few calories and high water content can help you lose weight.

Research shows how much you eat and whether you feel full afterward depends more on the size of a portion — its volume — than on the amount of calories, or energy. Make a small portion of food look larger, and you'll eat less yet feel fuller. This optical illusion can be a dieter's best friend. By tricking your eyes, and therefore your stomach, you can naturally eat less without feeling deprived.

High-water, low-calorie, nutrient-rich foods like mung bean sprouts are perfect accomplices in your weight-loss efforts. Add a cup of sprouts to your next stir-fry, soup, or casserole. Mound them on a sandwich in place of lettuce, or sprinkle them in salads for crunchy variety.

Cook's corner

- When shopping for raw sprouts, look for crisp ones with firm, white shoots. Don't buy musty-smelling, dark, or slimy sprouts.

- For the most flavor and nutrition, use them as soon as possible. You can refrigerate mung bean sprouts in a vegetable crisper or plastic bag up to four days. Rinsing them under cold water daily may extend their life. Wash again and trim off the roots just before serving.

- Add raw sprouts to salads, sandwiches, burgers, and tacos, or boil them in soups. If you stir-fry them, toss them in last and cook for no more than 30 seconds to avoid wilting.

Stay safe while eating sprouts

In 2006, alfalfa sprouts were named one of the seven riskiest foods by the Centers for Disease Control. The dangerous secret they sometimes harbor? Harmful bacteria such as *E. coli* and *Salmonella*.

Alfalfa sprouts aren't the only ones, either. Mung bean, radish, cress, clover, and other sprouts can all carry these bad bugs. One of the biggest reasons sprouts are a potential source of food poisoning — people usually eat them raw. Cooking kills most harmful bugs.

Most healthy adults will feel sick for a few days before fighting off the bug. But the elderly, children, and people with weak immune systems can become seriously ill from eating contaminated sprouts. Luckily, you can take a few simple steps to protect yourself.

Ask restaurants to "hold the raw sprouts" on sandwiches and salads.

- Cook your sprouts. Boil or stir-fry sprouts before eating, but do it thoroughly. Light cooking won't destroy all the bacteria. Mung bean sprouts are the only ones sturdy enough to stir-fry.

- Don't grow your own sprouts. They won't be any safer than store-bought sprouts. Indeed, they may be more dangerous. If the beans you buy to sprout are already contaminated, then your sprouts will be, too, no matter how clean the growing conditions. Professional growers take extra steps to kill germs on seeds before they sprout. Unfortunately, you don't have the same chemical methods at home.

Contact your doctor immediately if you eat sprouts and develop diarrhea, nausea, stomach cramps, or a fever. These are typical signs of food poisoning.

Soybeans

■ ■ ■ ■ ■ ■ ■ ■ ■ ■ ■ ■ ■ ■

Discover the joys of soy

Soybeans pack more protein than beef and more calcium than milk. In fact, scientists rate soybean protein equal to meat in quality, partly because soybeans provide complete protein. Since they cost less, they make an inexpensive alternative to meat-based meals without skimping on nutrition.

Plus, soybeans contain four and a half times more polyunsaturated than saturated fats, which will make your heart happy. Their goodness doesn't stop there, though. They're a rich source of monounsaturated fats, fiber, iron, phosphorous manganese, and unique plant compounds called isoflavones.

In the United States, soybeans are a bigger cash crop than corn or wheat, and the U.S. produces more soybeans than any country in the world. Maybe that's because these beans are so versatile. They're made into everything from vegetable oil, animal feed, and newspaper ink to dried beans, soy milk, and tofu.

Surefire way to build better bones. The hormone estrogen helps keep your bones strong. After menopause, women's estrogen levels drop sharply, and bones become thinner and more likely to break. Experts now say estrogen replacement therapy is too risky to take just for bone strength. Soybeans may fill the

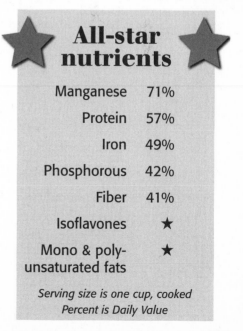

All-star nutrients

Manganese	71%
Protein	57%
Iron	49%
Phosphorous	42%
Fiber	41%
Isoflavones	★
Mono & poly-unsaturated fats	★

Serving size is one cup, cooked
Percent is Daily Value

gap with phytochemicals known as isoflavones. Also called phytoestrogens, these natural plant compounds act similar to estrogen in your body.

In a study of almost 400 post-menopausal women with osteopenia, half took a supplement of calcium and vitamin D and half took a supplement containing calcium, vitamin D, and 54 milligrams (mg) of a soy isoflavone called genistein. After two years, the genistein group had boosted their bone density, not just maintained it. Isoflavones seem to encourage your body to build new bone and keep it from breaking down old bone, adding to your bottom-line bone density.

Experts warn that soy supplements may not be safe to take long term. Soy foods, on the other hand, enjoy a strong safety record. After all, they've been a staple of Asian diets for centuries. A cup of soy milk with breakfast, another with lunch, and a half cup of boiled soybeans with dinner give you 58 mg of genistein. See *Cook's corner* at the end of this chapter for more ways to enjoy soy.

■ ■ ■ ■ ■ **Boost the benefits** ■ ■ ■ ■ ■

The American Heart Association says replacing fatty, high-cholesterol animal foods with soy alternatives may benefit your heart. Consider these substitutions:

- tofu or edamame in place of red meat

- soybean-based butter instead of regular butter

- soy burgers for hamburgers

Fiber may help you absorb more phytoestrogens, so eat soybeans or other soy products alongside fiber-rich foods. Soy contains protein, so people with sensitive food allergies may need to avoid it.

Ease the flush of menopause. More than half of women suffer hot flashes during menopause and for years afterward. With questions about the safety of hormone replacement therapy, soybeans may offer hope for women fed up with sleepless nights and embarrassing flushes.

Have heart: the scoop on soy

The American Heart Association (AHA) says soy protein supplements do little to prevent cardiovascular diseases (CVD). They don't seem to boost your good HDL cholesterol, lower triglycerides, or reduce high blood pressure. Plus, you would need to take huge amounts of soy protein to lower your cholesterol only a few points, which might not be safe long-term.

Soybeans, however, are a different matter. The AHA says soy foods such as tofu, soybeans, soy nuts, and soy burgers may help your heart. Soy foods provide more than just protein. They're loaded with polyunsaturated fats, fiber, vitamins, and minerals, and are low in saturated fat. Replacing high-fat, high-cholesterol animal foods with soy substitutes may, indeed, make your heart sing.

Scientists suspect a drop in estrogen levels leads to lower amounts of endorphins in your brain. This makes your body release extra brain chemicals called serotonin and epinephrine, which throws off your internal thermostat. Your body thinks it is overheating, so it goes to extremes trying to let off the "extra" heat.

The isoflavones in soybeans may help fill the void left by falling estrogen levels. Results are mixed but suggest soy may make hot flashes less frequent and severe for women in the early stages of menopause who have mild to moderate hot flashes. Soy does not seem to improve hot flashes in women who have had breast cancer.

Go nuts to guard your heart. Replacing some of the animal protein in your diet with plant protein from soybeans could be your body's first line of defense against stroke, high cholesterol, and heart and liver damage.

That's because snacking on crunchy soy nuts fights metabolic syndrome, a group of symptoms including high blood pressure, low HDL cholesterol, high triglycerides, belly fat obesity, and prediabetes or diabetes that, put together, sends your risk of heart disease, diabetes, and stroke skyrocketing. In 42 women with metabolic syndrome, eating an ounce of soy nuts in place of red meat for eight weeks lowered bad LDL cholesterol and fasting blood sugar levels, plus improved their insulin resistance. In fact, soy nuts had a much greater impact on all these numbers than taking soy protein supplements. Other research shows soy protein helps protect your liver from alcohol damage.

Experts say soy nuts, flavorful and roasted like peanuts, provide a whole package of nutrients that benefit your body, such as unsaturated fats and isoflavones, not just protein. Look for them in the health food section of your supermarket.

Seed sweeps away cholesterol

The guar plant, an important legume in India, yields a cluster bean called the guar seed. Grind these seeds into powder, and you get guar gum — an excellent thickener similar to cornstarch. Food manufacturers do just that, adding guar gum to ice cream, salad dressing, instant noodles, dough, batter, snack foods, gravies, beverages, and even fake whipped cream. You probably eat foods that contain it every day.

That's good news for your heart, because this little seed sweeps artery-clogging cholesterol right out of your system. Guar gum is 75 percent soluble fiber, the kind that traps cholesterol and carries it out with your stool. Eating foods made with guar gum could help lower your total cholesterol. Just be sure to choose those low in saturated and trans fats and rich in other healthy nutrients.

Lose weight and trim body fat. Meeting more of your protein needs with soybeans could help you trim body fat, lose more weight, feel fuller after meals, improve insulin resistance, lower the amount of fat your body tends to store, plus keep plaque from building up in your arteries.

For any weight-loss plan to work, you need to cut excess calories from your diet. Fitting soy foods into your eating plan may give you an added boost. In one study, obese adults cut calories and replaced all animal protein — from sources like meat, chicken, and dairy — with soy protein. They lost more weight and body fat and saw a bigger drop in total and LDL cholesterol than obese people who cut calories but kept eating animal protein.

A second, small study in post-menopausal women found soy protein kept them from packing on belly fat, compared to their peers who ate the same calories but didn't get soy.

Strengthen cancer defenses naturally. Soy-based foods like tofu and miso soup may protect men from localized prostate cancer. The results of a study on more than 40,000 Japanese men suggest the isoflavones in soy foods like miso soup and tofu prevent the growth of localized prostate tumors in men over age 60. However, they may not protect younger men against the early stages of prostate cancer.

Questions still linger about soy for breast cancer. Experts think eating soy foods during your teenage years may lower your risk of breast cancer later in life, but findings in adults aren't so clear. Some studies suggest soy phytoestrogens help prevent breast cancer, while other studies suggest they contribute to it. A recent German review concluded that long-term use of isoflavone supplements is risky for menopausal women. The bottom line — you can safely enjoy soy foods as part of a balanced diet, but avoid soy supplements, especially if you take the breast-cancer drug tamoxifen.

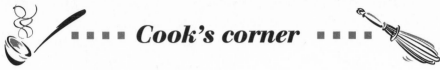

Cook's corner

Soy nuts can be hard to find in grocery stores, but making your own is a snap.

- Soak dried soybeans for eight hours. Drain and spread them on oiled cookie sheets.

- Roast at 350 degrees for around 30 minutes, stirring occasionally. Remove when they are golden brown.

Season your soy nuts with your favorite flavors — cayenne pepper, Cajun seasonings, garlic salt, or plain salt. Coarsely grind them to replace bacon bits in salads.

Tofu, on the other hand, is readily available in most supermarkets. It has little flavor on its own but easily absorbs the flavor of juices and marinades. Liquefy soft tofu in a blender and use in place of sour cream, yogurt, or soft cheeses. You can sauté, braise, fry, or grill firm tofu in place of meat in dishes.

Nuts & Seeds: small but mighty

Almonds

■ ■ ■ ■ ■ ■ ■ ■ ■ ■ ■ ■ ■

Add joy to your life with a nut-ritious treat

Sometimes you feel like a nut. When that craving strikes, go with it. Although nuts have a reputation of being fatty and loaded with calories, they actually do great things for your body. Some nuts — like almonds and walnuts — give you fiber, protein, healthy monounsaturated fats, vitamins, and minerals. What's more, the Food and Drug Administration allows nut growers to boast that eating certain nuts may lower your risk of heart disease.

Almonds got their start in Asia, but the Romans called them the "Greek nut." By the time hopeful miners rushed to find gold in California, almonds were already there. In fact, most of the U.S. crop is still grown in California.

Along with a healthy dose of monounsaturated fats, almonds have vitamin E and minerals, like copper, magnesium, and manganese. Add them to home-baked goods, sprinkle them on salads, or munch them straight from the package.

Sweet almonds are the kind you eat, while bitter almonds are used to make almond oil for flavoring and cosmetics.

Keep a lid on blood sugar. People with diabetes struggle to keep their blood sugar from getting too high. Eating almonds may help keep it in check. Researchers tested this theory on people who did not have diabetes, feeding them

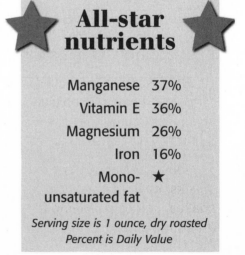

All-star nutrients

Manganese	37%
Vitamin E	36%
Magnesium	26%
Iron	16%
Mono-unsaturated fat	★

Serving size is 1 ounce, dry roasted
Percent is Daily Value

meals that were guaranteed to raise their blood sugar, like white bread, white rice, and mashed potatoes. Sure enough, blood sugar went up.

Then the researchers tried similar meals — but this time they added either 1, 2, or 3 ounces of almonds. Again, the meal-eaters' blood sugar rose, but not as much. In fact, people who ate the most almonds had the smallest jump in blood sugar.

Experts believe the monounsaturated fats in almonds keep blood sugar from rising too quickly after you eat. If you have type 2 diabetes, they recommend eating more nuts and fewer carbohydrates to get this benefit — and to lower your triglycerides. The healthy fats in almonds are also known to lower cholesterol, while the fiber may help control your blood sugar, reduce your weight, and keep your heart healthy.

People who don't have diabetes may even ward off the disease by eating nuts several times a week. But don't go nutty in your almond eating. Three ounces of dry-roasted almonds have a whopping 500 calories.

Cut your cholesterol without medication. Almonds are tasty, popular, and they may help lower your cholesterol. That's what scientists found at a cardiac research center in California. They studied a group of men and women with high cholesterol for four weeks, recording what they ate and how their cholesterol levels changed. Some of the people

---

Add variety with high-protein hemp

Heard about hemp? It's the latest fashion in food.

Nutty-tasting hempseeds have loads of good-quality protein, and hemp oil boasts of heart-healthy omega-3 fatty acids. You'll also get the benefits of vitamin E; fiber; and minerals like magnesium, iron, and potassium.

You can buy seeds or powder to sprinkle on cereal or snacks, or seek out hemp in foods like granola bars, bread, shakes, and chips. Hemp fiber is also used in clothing, soap, and other products.

added 100 grams of raw, unblanched almonds to their diet every day. Others added olive oil or butter, along with cheese and crackers.

At the end of the study, the people who ate almonds every day had lowered their cholesterol from an average of 251 to 222 mg/dL. That's nearly a 30-point drop in cholesterol — no drugs required. Experts think it's the monounsaturated fatty acids in almonds and some other nuts that help lower cholesterol.

You'd need to eat a lot of almonds to equal what the people in the study ate — about two-thirds of a cup every day. But even a smaller amount of almonds may help you lower your cholesterol by 20 points.

■ ■ ■ ■ ■ **Boost the benefits** ■ ■ ■ ■ ■

Don't take a good nut and turn it bad. Almonds are rich in healthy fats, mostly monounsaturated fat, like olive oil. When almonds are roasted in coconut or palm oil, they gain a lot of unhealthy saturated fat — along with extra calories. So choose raw or dry roasted almonds instead of oil roasted. Your heart and your waistline will thank you.

Maintain a healthy brain. Diseases that affect your memory, like Alzheimer's disease, and how your brain controls your body, like Parkinson's disease, are more common as you age.

Vitamin E might play a role in keeping your brain healthy. It works as an antioxidant to clean up free radicals, which roam the body damaging cells. Researchers think antioxidants in your brain may protect cells from damage that can cause age-related problems. One study of more than 120,000 men and women found those who got the most vitamin E from the food they ate had less chance of developing Parkinson's disease. People who took vitamin E supplements during the study didn't get this protection.

Still, other research shows getting enough vitamin E may also lower your risk of developing Alzheimer's disease. But not all studies agree on what vitamin E does, and experts know both diseases are affected by heredity. To increase your protection, dig into a can of almonds. One ounce of these dry-roasted treats has more than a third of the vitamin E you need every day.

Tell arthritis to take a hike. Wearing a copper bracelet to fight arthritis pain won't help, but getting more copper in your diet could offer relief. Research on animals shows that copper supplements may slow the progress of arthritis. You also need the essential mineral copper to build bone and other connective tissue. If you don't get enough copper, you may be at risk of breaking a bone or developing osteoporosis. Fend off arthritis and keep your bones strong with a daily handful of almonds, a great source of copper.

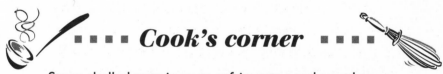

■ ■ ■ ■ *Cook's corner* ■ ■ ■ ■

Store shelled nuts in your refrigerator to keep them from going rancid.

If you're buying nuts for baking, keep these quantities in mind.

- One pound almonds in the shell will yield one-and-a-half to two cups after shelling.

- One pound shelled almonds equals three to three-and-a-half cups whole almonds or four cups slivered almonds.

When you are selecting nuts in the shell, pick those that feel heavy for their size and are clean and free of mold.

Fenugreek

■ ■ ■ ■ ■ ■ ■ ■ ■ ■ ■ ■ ■ ■ ■

Funny-sounding seed offers serious benefits

Is it a spice? A vegetable? A seed? Fenugreek could be all three, depending on what part of the plant you pick and how you use it. It's a clover-like plant with seedpods, belonging to the bean family. Fenugreek is an ancient medicinal herb, with a variety of alleged healing powers. Moroccan women still use fenugreek to enhance their appetites, and other people try the herb to treat hair loss or relieve digestive complaints.

Modern scientists are looking at fenugreek as a possible remedy for stomach ulcers, colon cancer, high cholesterol, and high blood sugar.

This little seed with the funny name can boast about fiber; high-quality protein, and minerals like iron, manganese, and copper. You can eat it in Indian curry, add the seeds to an entree, or take it in capsules.

Bring down high blood sugar. People with diabetes wage a constant battle against high blood sugar. Although taking drugs and watching what you eat can help, fenugreek — a traditional remedy for diabetes — might be another powerful weapon.

Many studies show fenugreek can lower high blood sugar in people with diabetes. Experts once thought trigonelline, a natural chemical in fenugreek, lowered blood sugar. But they've managed to break down fenugreek into its components to figure out what's doing the trick. Now they think the high level of fiber should get the

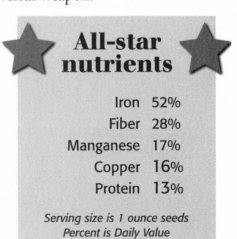

All-star nutrients

Iron	52%
Fiber	28%
Manganese	17%
Copper	16%
Protein	13%

Serving size is 1 ounce seeds
Percent is Daily Value

credit. Fenugreek seeds are about 52 percent fiber. Their soluble fiber slows digestion, making it take longer for sugar to get into your blood. Some experts suggest 1 to 2 ounces of fenugreek seeds daily should help.

■ ■ ■ ■ ■ **Boost the benefits** ■ ■ ■ ■ ■

Fenugreek helps make Indian curry spicy. It has a strong odor and bittersweet flavor. You can enjoy fenugreek even if you can't take the heat of a traditional curry. Instead, use the roasted seeds to add flavor to soups, vegetables, cheese, pickles, and simmered dishes. Or try letting the seeds sprout and making a salad. Some people enjoy tea made from fenugreek leaves or seeds.

Researchers are also looking into whether fenugreek seeds can lower high cholesterol. So far, studies look promising, but more research is needed.

■ ■ ■ ■ *Cook's corner* ■ ■ ■ ■

Fenugreek seeds are available whole, ground, crushed, sprouted, or dried. They're more flavorful after they're roasted and ground. In fact, roasting the seeds helps remove the natural bitter flavor. You can also buy fenugreek extract in a liquid or spray, poultice, capsules, tablets, and tea.

For fresher taste, try grinding your own fenugreek seeds. You'll need a special poppy seed grinder for this job. The seeds are too hard to grind using a mortar and pestle. Store the seeds in an airtight container in a cool, dry, dark place.

Flaxseed

■ ■ ■ ■ ■ ■ ■ ■ ■ ■ ■ ■ ■

Ancient crop offers amazing seeds and oil

Blonde girls in fairy tales are often called "flaxen-haired," referring to their golden locks. In fact, flaxseed, also called linseed, grows in both yellow and reddish-brown varieties. It's an ancient crop used to make linen fabric, linseed oil for linoleum and oilcloth, and flaxseed and flaxseed oil for people and animals to eat.

Cherokee legend has it that flaxseed oil brings good health because it contains energy caught from the sun. No matter the source, flaxseed and oil are great sources of vitamins and minerals, like thiamin and manganese, and heart-healthy omega-3 fatty acids. Lignans, natural plant chemicals in flaxseeds, may help prevent some kinds of cancer. Some people eat flaxseed — a good source of fiber — to help their digestion, while others believe the oil can make their hair healthy and treat dandruff.

Flaxseed may not be as common as other seeds, but they're well worth bringing to the table. They're gluten-free, so people with celiac disease or other gluten sensitivities can eat them. They add a hearty, nutty taste to breads and cereals. And who knows — they just may make you feel as healthy and happy as any fairy tale princess.

Curb cholesterol with tough tactics. Flaxseed has three heavy hitters when it comes to lowering high cholesterol — soluble fiber, alpha-linolenic acid (ALA), and

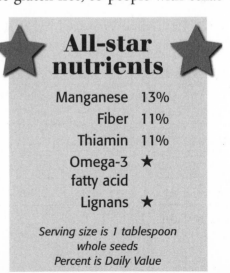

All-star nutrients

Manganese	13%
Fiber	11%
Thiamin	11%
Omega-3 fatty acid	★
Lignans	★

Serving size is 1 tablespoon whole seeds
Percent is Daily Value

Break out of your rut
with nut butters

Longtime habits lead many people to eat the same foods — like peanut butter — year after year. Why not add some pizzazz to your meals with a variety of nut butters and oils. You'll find tasty butters made of almonds, hazelnuts, macadamia nuts, cashews, and sunflower seeds. Just be sure to check the label for hydrogenated oils on the ingredients list. Some nut butters — peanut butter included — have unhealthy trans fats added to make them smoother and last longer. Also, if a nut butter has an added flavor, like chocolate, it's probably high in sugar. Remember — even the purest nut butters are still rich in calories, so stick to a 2-tablespoon serving.

Check out the many different oils made from nuts and seeds. Decide how you'll be using an oil so you'll know which one to pick. Each type has a different smoke point, or temperature where it starts to burn. You should use an oil with a high smoke point for higher temperature cooking, like frying. For the healthiest choice, pick an oil with less saturated fat.

Oil (100 grams)	Saturated fat (grams)	Smoke point (degrees Fahrenheit)	Best uses
canola oil (rapeseed)	7	460	baking, broiling
flaxseed oil	9	225	salad dressing
peanut oil	17	425	all
sunflower oil	10	410–425	cooking, table use
walnut oil	9	325–400	salad dressing

lignans. Here's what each does to keep your bad LDL cholesterol down and your blood flowing smoothly.

- Soluble fiber, the kind that forms a gooey gel in water, acts like a sponge. It absorbs cholesterol and excretes it as waste, which helps lower your cholesterol level. Oatmeal has a great reputation for providing lots of soluble fiber, and flaxseed ranks in the same category. In fact, one tablespoon of flaxseed has nearly as much soluble fiber as one-third cup of dry oatmeal.

- The essential fatty acid ALA, another type of omega-3 fatty acid, helps stop inflammation, keeps blood cells from clumping together, lowers your blood pressure, and improves cholesterol levels. In one study, eating two to six tablespoons of ground flaxseed every day for four weeks brought down bad LDL — without changing the good HDL. Flaxseed is the top food source for ALA.

- Lignans are plant chemicals that can do a lot for your body. Researchers are looking at how they may fight cancer and work as antioxidants to clean up free radicals. Some research shows lignans may lower LDL and total cholesterol, while they raise HDL. One study found men who ate the most lignans had the lowest risk for heart disease.

ALA, soluble fiber, and lignans work together, so it's hard to tell exactly how each part of flaxseed is really doing the trick. Even without knowing how, you may be able to lower your cholesterol by eating between one and five tablespoons of flaxseed a day.

Do battle against breast and prostate cancer. Some of the same ingredients in flaxseed that help it fight high cholesterol also make it a winner against some cancers. The lignans, or plant chemicals, in flaxseed work against the estrogen your body makes. Estrogen encourages certain cancers, like breast cancer, to grow.

Experts think lignans block estrogen, which slows tumor growth or stops them from forming. In fact, lignans work like the cancer drug tamoxifen. One study of older women with breast cancer found those who ate a flaxseed muffin every day for about 35 days had slower tumor growth. In addition, flaxseed has lots of fiber, which may also lower your chances of getting breast cancer.

It's not clear how the lignans in flaxseed affect prostate cancer, another cancer affected by hormones. Some experts worry lignans in high doses may actually encourage prostate tumors to develop. But a recent study of men with prostate cancer found those who ate three tablespoons of flaxseed every day had slower tumor growth. Ask your doctor for advice on taking flaxseed to prevent or treat prostate or breast cancer.

■ ■ ■ ■ ■ **Boost the benefits** ■ ■ ■ ■ ■

You can buy whole flaxseed to sprinkle on salads, cereals, or stir-fry dishes, while ground flaxseed works well in baked recipes. Both are good sources of fiber, protein, and alpha-linolenic acid, a healthy omega-3 fatty acid. But a tablespoon of whole seeds has more of all three of these nutrients than a tablespoon of ground flaxseed, plus whole seeds stay fresh longer in your pantry. If you eat flaxseeds whole, be sure to chew them well. Otherwise, they'll pass through your digestive system intact, and you'll miss out on the nutrients.

Take a bite out of menopause. Hot flashes, night sweats, sleeplessness, mood swings — the "change" can make being a woman no fun. Many women shy away from taking hormone-replacement therapy (HRT) for their menopausal symptoms because of serious side effects. Flaxseed might be a safe alternative to drugs and help you get through the change more comfortably.

Flaxseed contains lignans — plant chemicals that work like your body's own estrogen but in a weaker form. Researchers have found eating flaxseed every day may reduce hot flashes and other signs of menopause. In one study, women who ate 40 grams — about four tablespoons — of ground flaxseed every day for several months got as much relief as women who took HRT. Not all studies on flaxseed and menopause have been so positive, but it probably won't hurt to add a little flaxseed to your diet.

Lube your joints to lessen arthritis pain. The fats in flaxseed and flaxseed oil may also help your aching joints. These omega-3 fatty acids, like the kind in fish oil, keep down the inflammation that can cause arthritis pain and may even protect your cartilage from breaking down. One study found women who ate the most omega-3 fatty acids had the least risk of developing rheumatoid arthritis. Researchers believe omega-3s from flaxseed work the same way as those in fish oil. Flaxseed oil is made of more than half omega-3 fatty acids, and you can buy it by the bottle or in capsules.

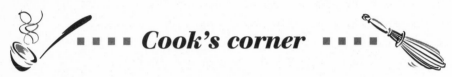

■ ■ ■ ■ *Cook's corner* ■ ■ ■ ■

Foods with flaxseed crowd the grocery shelves, from cereals, waffles, and yogurt to caramel chews and soy drinks. Try flaxseed for lunch or dinner in pasta, bread, or a frozen dessert, and fix yourself a snack of flaxseed-added popcorn.

Flaxseed won't stay good forever. Follow these tips for safe storage and cooking.

- Whole flaxseed stays fresh at room temperature for a year or more, while ground flaxseed stays good for four months. Keep them both in the refrigerator or freezer, and they'll be fresh even longer.

- Store an unopened bottle of flaxseed oil at room temperature. After it's opened, store it in the refrigerator and use it within six weeks.

- Flaxseed oil is best used cool, like in salad dressing or yogurt. You can stir-fry lightly using flaxseed oil, but don't get it too hot. Keep the temperature lower than 300 degrees Fahrenheit — too cool for frying.

Pistachios

Go green for healthy snacking

In ancient Assyria, the Queen of Sheba was so fond of pistachios she kept the country's entire harvest for herself and her royal household. There's a lot to like about this tiny, tasty nut. It has a delicate, sweet flavor that works well in both desserts and main dishes. The thin shell opens by itself, so it's not a tough nut to crack. Many people remember pistachios by their color — the nuts are naturally pale green, while processors often dye the shells red to hide spots.

Pistachios make for a guilt-free snack. You can eat 50 pistachios and only take in about 160 calories. Even better, you're also getting fiber, vitamin B6, phytosterols to fight high cholesterol, healthy monounsaturated fat, and minerals like manganese and potassium. All these qualities make pistachios a treat fit for a queen.

Nutty control for high cholesterol. Oatmeal is not the only food that can help keep your cholesterol in check. Pistachios are rich in phytosterols, plant chemicals similar to your body's cholesterol. They work in your intestines to block cholesterol in food from being absorbed. This means lower cholesterol. New analysis of popular snack foods shows pistachios and sunflower seeds contain the most phytosterols — about three times as much as the lowly Brazil nut.

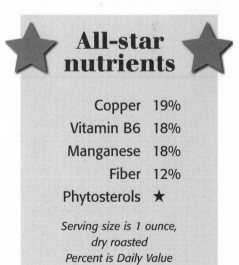

All-star nutrients

Copper	19%
Vitamin B6	18%
Manganese	18%
Fiber	12%
Phytosterols	★

Serving size is 1 ounce, dry roasted
Percent is Daily Value

■ ■ ■ ■ ■ **Boost the benefits** ■ ■ ■ ■ ■

As nuts go, pistachios are high in potassium — a winner if you're keeping an eye on your blood pressure. But pick your pistachios wisely if you're on a low-sodium diet.

Dry-roasted, salted pistachios have 114 milligrams (mg) of sodium in 1 ounce, or about 49 nuts. Instead, select the unsalted variety, with just 3 mg of sodium. Or even better, try raw pistachios, which have no sodium at all and are a bit lower in calories.

Just how powerful are pistachios? Several studies show they work to bring cholesterol levels back into balance.

- Men and women with healthy cholesterol levels were divided into two groups. People in one group continued their regular diet, while those in the other group got 20 percent of their daily calories from pistachios for three weeks. Total cholesterol went down and good HDL cholesterol went up for the pistachio eaters.

- A group of 28 people with high cholesterol ate either 3 ounces or 1 1/2 ounces a day of pistachios. Both groups showed lower levels of total cholesterol and LDL cholesterol after four weeks, but those who ate the most pistachios had the greatest improvement.

- Fifteen people with high cholesterol ate 2 to 3 ounces of pistachios every day. After four weeks, most people had lower total cholesterol and LDL cholesterol — but higher HDL cholesterol.

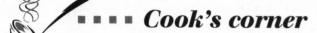

Cook's corner

Pistachio shells open naturally as they mature. If you find one that hasn't opened on its own, don't bother prying it open. The nut inside won't be good anyway.

Because the shells open naturally, pistachios don't last as long as many other nuts. If you buy shelled pistachios, select some that come vacuum-packed in glass jars or cans to get the freshest nuts.

Store pistachios in an airtight container. You can keep unshelled pistachios for three months in the refrigerator or for a year in the freezer. But don't freeze shelled pistachios.

Nutty way to take off extra pounds

Want to lose weight? Go nuts. Studies show adding nuts to your diet won't make you gain weight, and you may even lose some pounds. Experts think that's because of the unsaturated fats in nuts like walnuts, almonds, peanuts, and pine nuts. These fats trigger your body to make appetite-blocking hormones, which tell your brain you're full. So chow down on a handful of nuts about 20 minutes before a meal, and you won't overdo it.

New label rules crack down on nut allergies

Food allergies are not just for kids. About 3 million Americans are allergic to peanuts and tree nuts, like walnuts, cashews, and almonds. Peanuts are the best-known allergy, but cashews can cause more severe reactions. If you eat a food you're allergic to, you may suffer from itching, nausea, or breathing problems. A severe allergic reaction, called anaphylactic shock, can kill.

Since 2006, the Food Allergen Labeling and Consumer Protection Act (FALCPA) requires labels to show whether the product includes milk, eggs, fish, crustacean shellfish, peanuts, tree nuts, wheat, and soybeans — the most common troublemakers. The label should show the word "contains" with the problem food, or it should include that food on the ingredients list.

Take these steps to avoid an allergic reaction.

- Check the label with every purchase. Older packages may still be on the shelves — even after FALCPA.

- Remember that some foods, including meat, poultry, vegetables, fruits, and alcoholic beverages, are exempt from FALCPA rules.

- When you dine out, tell your server or the person preparing the food how serious your allergy is. Don't let impatient staff brush off your questions about food ingredients.

- Kiss with care. Studies show allergens stay in the saliva of people who eat peanuts for quite a while — even if they brush their teeth or chew gum. If you're allergic to peanuts, kissing that person exposes you to the peanuts. Ask your honey to stay away from the food you're allergic to, or wait a few hours before you get close.

Researchers are working on vaccines that could make you less sensitive to problem foods.

Sunflower seeds

■■■■■■■■■■■■■■■■■■■■■■■■■■■

Tasty kernels not just for the birds

Painter Vincent van Gogh loved to paint sunflowers, and people in Kansas, the sunflower state, love to grow them. Poets have called these happy flowers "restless" and "light-enchanted sunflowers," thinking they turn their faces to follow the sun. They don't — although their name suggests it.

People once grew sunflower plants around their houses to ward off disease. That trick probably won't work, but eating the seeds may bring you good health. Sunflower seeds have oodles of vitamin E, plenty of fiber, and minerals like phosphorous and copper. They're also packed with phytosterols to lower your cholesterol. As snack foods go, sunflower seeds are a smart choice.

Shield your heart with vitamin E. Sunflower seeds have several heart-healthy ingredients, including phytosterols and unsaturated fats. And 1 ounce of dry-roasted sunflower seeds gives you more than a third of the vitamin E you need every day.

What's so great about vitamin E? It's an antioxidant, so it helps protect your cells against free-radical damage. Many studies have been done to find out if vitamin E can help your heart. Some show it may prevent heart attacks and keep heart disease from getting worse. Other research suggests

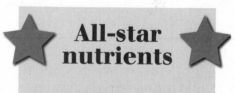

All-star nutrients

Vitamin E	37%
Phosphorous	32%
Copper	26%
Fiber	12%
Phytosterols	★

Serving size is 1 ounce
Percent is Daily Value

taking vitamin E supplements may not help and may even raise your risk of heart failure and death.

To be safe, get your vitamin E from food instead of supplements. Some experts think the type of vitamin E in sunflower seeds and olive oil, alpha-tocopherol, is safer than the kind in corn and soybeans, gamma-tocopherol.

■ ■ ■ ■ ■ **Boost the benefits** ■ ■ ■ ■ ■

You can buy sunflower seeds raw or roasted, in the shell or out, and with or without salt. Roasted seeds often have added fat and preservatives, so make a healthy batch at home. Put raw seeds on a baking sheet and roast them in the oven for about 10 minutes at 200 degrees Fahrenheit, stirring often. For a salty flavor, spray with a bit of oil and season with salt.

Send hay fever packing. Sunflower seeds are an old folk remedy for baldness, headaches, sunstroke, lung ailments, and other illnesses. Those uses may be doubtful, but the generous supply of vitamin E in these tiny seeds may make them a good tonic for your seasonal sneezing and wheezing.

Some people know spring is in the air when their eyes start watering and their noses get runny. That's from breathing in certain kinds of plant pollen. Vitamin E is an antioxidant, so it helps fight inflammation. Researchers in Germany wanted to find out whether the foods people eat have an effect on hay fever. They surveyed the eating habits of more than 1,500 people — some with hay fever, some without. People who tended to get more vitamin E in their diets had less hay fever.

Other researchers tested vitamin E supplements for hay fever symptoms. Half the people in the study took 800 milligrams of vitamin E supplements each day, while the other half took a placebo, or sugar pill. They all continued to take their usual anti-allergy medications during the study. People in the vitamin E group reported less trouble with a runny nose but no change in their itchy, watery eyes.

It's best to get your vitamin E from food instead of supplements. One reason is that about half the substances in vitamin E pills are not active. So you'd need to take twice as much to get the same effect as a similar amount of vitamin E from food. Along with sunflower seeds, good sources of vitamin E include peanuts, almonds, olive oil, and avocados.

▪ ▪ ▪ ▪ *Cook's corner* ▪ ▪ ▪ ▪

Add more of sunflower seeds' benefits to your diet with sunflower oil. It's made from a different kind of seeds than the ones you snack on, but it's still high in vitamin E. Sunflower oil has lots of good-for-you unsaturated fats, and you can use it for cooking or in salad dressings. It also stays fresh longer than some other plant oils.

Walnuts

■ ■ ■ ■ ■ ■ ■ ■ ■ ■ ■

Go nuts to guard your heart and mind

Roman legend has it that walnuts brought good health and fertility, while they scared away disease. Folk medicine used walnuts to treat earache, toothache, warts, ringworm, poison ivy, boils, arthritis, and constipation.

Much of those claims may be only legend, but walnuts truly are a treat for your heart. They're about 60 percent fat, most of it healthy monounsaturated fat. This type of fat helps keep your cholesterol and blood pressure down and your arteries clear. These little nuggets of nutrition are also high in protein, minerals like copper and manganese, and antioxidants like glutathione. Their healthy fats make them good food for your brain, helping to protect your memory into old age.

So even though walnuts — especially black walnuts — can be tough nuts to crack, don't leave them out of your healthy diet. Toss them on a Waldorf salad, bake them into a fruit cake, mix them into ice cream, or eat them straight from the shell — walnuts are a nutritional powerhouse.

Nibble your way to a healthy heart. Nuts are good for your heart, and walnuts lead the pack. The healthy fats in walnuts make them heart-helpers in several ways.

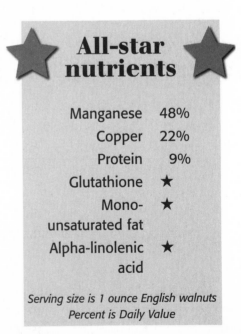

All-star nutrients

Manganese	48%
Copper	22%
Protein	9%
Glutathione	★
Mono-unsaturated fat	★
Alpha-linolenic acid	★

Serving size is 1 ounce English walnuts
Percent is Daily Value

- Bring down LDL cholesterol. Researchers tested a "walnut diet" on people with high cholesterol. Half the people in the study ate a typical Mediterranean diet, with olive oil as the main source of fat. The other half ate a similar diet but replaced most of the olive oil with fat from walnuts. They ate about eight to 11 fresh walnuts each day. Those on the walnut diet lowered their LDL cholesterol by more than 11 percent after six weeks — twice the improvement of those on the Mediterranean diet. The researchers think the fat in walnuts is what did the trick.

- Cap off high blood pressure. Eating foods high in omega-3 fatty acids, like fish, may lower your blood pressure. If you don't like fish, get your omega-3s from walnuts, flaxseed, canola oil, or soybean oil. These foods contain alpha-linolenic acid, another type of omega-3. Research shows people who eat more foods rich in omega-3s tend to have lower blood pressure than people who skip them.

- Say nuts to heart attacks. A large study of more than 43,000 people found those who ate more foods high in alpha-linolenic acid lowered their heart attack risk by 60 percent. Other research has shown similar results.

■ ■ ■ ■ ■ **Boost the benefits** ■ ■ ■ ■ ■

English walnuts and black walnuts are the most common of the many species of this nut. English, or Persian, walnuts are most commonly grown in California and sold for eating. English walnuts have thinner shells and more meat in each nut, but the black variety may be a better choice for good nutrition. They have less fat and more protein, fiber, and iron per cup.

Along with good fats, walnuts also give you glutathione. Your body uses this antioxidant to boost immunity and stop cell damage, possibly reducing your risk of heart disease and other health problems. Experts suggest you eat about a quarter to a third cup of walnuts every day, but avoid salted or honey-roasted nuts.

Crack down on memory loss. Most people think a bad memory is a natural sign of getting older. But some experts think you can keep your brain going strong as you age by eating certain fats — including the kind of fats in walnuts.

Researchers tested this theory by studying older people in Italy. The scientists checked out the diets of these healthy people, ages 65 to 84 years old. They also gave them tests to see how well they could remember and concentrate on mental tasks. The people who ate more monounsaturated fats — like the fat in walnuts — did better on the tests.

Scientists are also looking for a link between walnuts and Alzheimer's disease. A lab study showed walnut extract stopped the protein changes that occur in the brains of people with Alzheimer's disease. They're not sure exactly what part of the walnut extract stopped these changes, but they think it's a phytochemical, or natural plant chemical, in walnuts. More research may prove how walnuts can keep your brain sharp.

■ ■ ■ *Cook's corner* ■ ■ ■ ■

If you buy walnuts in the shell, you have the job of setting them free. Try this trick to make them easier to crack. Cover walnuts with water in a pan and bring to a boil. Remove them from heat and let sit for 15 minutes. Once the walnuts cool, your job will be easier.

Walnuts contain lots of fat, so store them carefully to keep them from going rancid.

- Store whole walnuts in a cool place, and they'll be good for months.

- Keep shelled walnuts in a sealed plastic bag in your freezer.

Anti-aging power from the sea

Crab

■ ■ ■ ■ ■ ■ ■

Crack open a shell full of goodness

You may not want crab grass in your lawn, but crab meat should be the prized jewel of your favorite meal. The versatile crab can be cooked many ways and used in a variety of dishes. In fact, writer H.L. Mencken quoted Baltimore lore that "crabs may be prepared in 50 ways and all of them are good."

Crack open its shell, and this ugly sea creature will reward you with some beautiful nutrients. It's loaded with vitamin B12 and important minerals like selenium, copper, and zinc. Crab is also a good bet if you're avoiding red meat. Eat a pair of dungeness crabs and you'll have all the protein you need for the day. Just don't rely on crabs or other shellfish for healthy omega-3 fatty acids. You'll find those in seafood like salmon and trout.

Cut your chances of colon cancer. A tasty crab dish may be your ticket to avoiding colon cancer. That's because crabs have lots of the important mineral selenium. It helps your body form enzymes to fight free radicals, tiny terrors that damage cells. Selenium also seems to boost your immunity so you can stay healthy.

Lots of research has found selenium can help keep tumors from growing in animals — including humans. In fact, some studies show that regions where people can get more selenium from their food also have lower rates of cancer. One

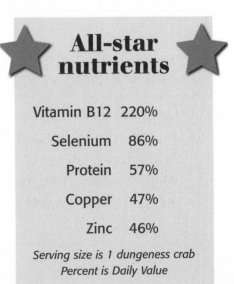

All-star nutrients

Vitamin B12	220%
Selenium	86%
Protein	57%
Copper	47%
Zinc	46%

Serving size is 1 dungeness crab
Percent is Daily Value

study checked how much selenium was in the blood of people who were having colonoscopies. The researchers found people with the most selenium had the fewest colon polyps — growths that sometimes become cancerous.

Watch your salt and cholesterol

Heart problems or high blood pressure may be forcing you to cut back on the sodium and cholesterol in your diet. Eat crab and shrimp with caution. Just one dungeness crab has 97 milligrams (mg) of cholesterol and 480 mg of sodium. That's one-third the cholesterol and one-fifth the sodium you should eat in an entire day.

Aside from Brazil nuts, crab meat is one of the best food sources of selenium. Eating just one dungeness crab gives you about 86 percent of the selenium you need in a day. At just 140 calories and more than half the protein you should get, that's a cancer-fighting bargain.

Zap pneumonia with zinc. Shellfish, including crab and oysters, along with red meat, are great sources of zinc. This important mineral helps your body's immune system fight off disease, but many older people don't get enough.

■ ■ ■ ■ ■ **Boost the benefits** ■ ■ ■ ■ ■

Lighten up traditional crab cakes. Cut the fat by using egg whites instead of mayonnaise to hold the cakes together. You can also sauté them in just a bit of oil rather than deep frying. For an added boost of healthful omega-3 fatty acids, cook the crab cakes in canola oil.

A recent study of older people in nursing homes tested whether zinc supplements could prevent pneumonia. For one year, residents took supplements of several vitamins and minerals, including zinc. Then researchers tested levels of zinc in the blood of everyone in the study. People with normal levels had fewer cases of pneumonia and took fewer antibiotics than those who were low in zinc. Residents with enough zinc also had less chance of dying during the study.

Research on children and zinc has shown similar results. So help sidestep pneumonia by adding some crab to your plate. Make it real crab though, since imitation crab is not a great source of zinc.

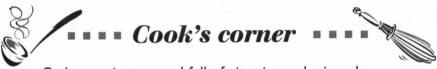

▪ ▪ ▪ ▪ *Cook's corner* ▪ ▪ ▪ ▪

Crab meat is tasty and full of vitamins and minerals, but buying it fresh can get expensive. For a cheaper substitute, you can use imitation crab meat in salads, crab cakes, and other recipes. A popular brand of imitation crab is about 50 cents an ounce compared to more than $1 an ounce for real crab meat.

But imitation crab meat is made from surimi, a kind of processed fish, so it doesn't have the nutritional benefits of real crab. With imitation crab, you'll get less cholesterol but also much less protein, vitamins, minerals, and omega-3 fats. Plus it has more than twice the sodium of real crab.

Benefits of eating fish outweigh the risks

You've probably heard about the dangers of eating fish and other seafood contaminated by mercury or polychlorinated biphenyls (PCBs). Mercury may cause nerve damage and heart problems, while high levels of PCBs are thought to cause cancer.

On the other hand, new guidelines recommend that all Americans eat fish two times a week. The omega-3 fatty acids in fatty fish — like salmon, sardines, tuna, and trout — may help you live a longer, healthier life. Research shows eating fish regularly may keep your heart healthy, ward off some forms of cancer, protect your vision, and keep your brain sharp. What should you do?

Eat fish — but be picky about what kind you choose. Women who are pregnant or nursing — and children — should choose carefully to avoid dangers to developing bodies. The table below outlines which fish are safest to eat most often. Check out the mercury calculator at *www.gotmercury.org* to see how safe your seafood-eating habits are. Experts say avoiding this great source of healthy omega-3 fatty acids is more harmful than eating it.

Safe — More than once a week	Relatively safe — Once a week	Risky — Once a month
salmon (farmed and wild)	canned tuna	tuna steaks
oysters	crab	red snapper
shrimp	cod	orange roughy
channel catfish (farmed)	mahi-mahi	pollock
rainbow trout (farmed)	haddock	halibut
flounder	whitefish	northern lobster
perch	herring	marlin
tilapia	spiny lobster	saltwater bass
clams		wild trout
scallops		grouper

Salmon

■ ■ ■ ■ ■ ■ ■ ■ ■ ■ ■

Get into the swim of healthy eating

The Salmon River in Idaho is known as the "river of no return." That's an odd name, because salmon do return to their birthplaces to spawn. If you're looking to return to healthful eating, salmon is a great choice.

Salmon, along with other fatty fish like trout and mackerel, contain healthy omega-3 fatty acids. They can help your heart, protect your brain as you age, prevent some kinds of cancers, and keep your eyesight sharp. Salmon also has lots of selenium and vitamins like niacin, vitamin B12, and vitamin B6. It's full of protein, so salmon makes a great substitute for red meat. Salmon is a better choice than some other types of seafood — including shark, swordfish, or tilefish — to avoid contaminants like mercury.

You can buy salmon fresh, frozen, smoked, dried, or canned. It's great as a steak, on a sandwich, in a salad — served either hot or cold. Switch to salmon and get many healthy returns.

Catch a batch of heart health. Some people take fish oil capsules to protect their hearts, but you can get a similar effect from eating fatty fish like salmon. The healthy omega-3 fatty acids in fish include eicosapentaenoic acid (EPA) and docosahexaenoic acid (DHA). They coat your arteries like a non-stick spray to keep your blood flowing smoothly.

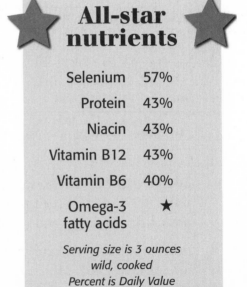

All-star nutrients

Selenium	57%
Protein	43%
Niacin	43%
Vitamin B12	43%
Vitamin B6	40%
Omega-3 fatty acids	★

Serving size is 3 ounces wild, cooked
Percent is Daily Value

■ ■ ■ ■ ■ Boost the benefits ■ ■ ■ ■ ■

Farmed salmon may be cheaper than wild, but it loses out when it comes to nutritional benefits. According to the U.S. Department of Agriculture, farm-raised salmon have fewer omega-3 fatty acids than wild salmon. Experts have also found higher levels of dangerous contaminants like polychlorinated biphenyls (PCBs) in farm-raised fish. The contaminants come from the food salmon eat in captivity. At high levels, PCBs and other poisons may cause cancer and problems with your brain and immune system. If you want the most benefits, stick with the wild varieties.

There's lots of evidence these healthy fats are good for your heart. Here's just a taste.

- A study in Japan of people with high cholesterol tested the effects of taking EPA supplements along with statins. After four to six years, people who took fish oil had fewer heart problems — including heart attacks, angina, and bypass operations — than those who only took statins. Omega-3 fatty acids also help keep your cholesterol in balance.

- Omega-3 fatty acids may protect you against heart disease. One study found that people with heart disease had less omega-3 in their bodies than people without heart disease. This may be due to the ability of some omega-3 fats to reduce inflammation, which can contribute to heart disease.

- People who get more omega-3 fatty acids in their diets tend to have lower blood pressure. Researchers found this link by looking at nearly 5,000 middle-aged men and women in the United States, Great Britain, China, and Japan.

- Other studies have found links between fats from fish and lower risks of stroke and heart rhythm problems.

To get these benefits, the American Heart Association urges everyone to eat fatty fish like salmon at least twice a week.

Reel in a healthier prostate. Salmon's EPA and DHA, the omega-3 fatty acids that help your heart, may also offer protection against prostate cancer.

Scientists have long noticed that groups of people who eat lots of fish, like Japanese and Eskimo men, tend to have fewer cases of prostate cancer. So they've been looking at men who eat traditional Western diets to see how eating fish might help.

A study of about 48,000 men found those who ate fatty fish more than three times a week had less risk of prostate cancer over 12 years. Eating shellfish or taking fish oil supplements didn't seem to help. In another study, men in Sweden who ate fatty fish like salmon at least once a week had fewer cases of prostate cancer than those who never ate fish.

Researchers think the omega-3 fats block natural body chemicals that help tumor cells grow. But other things could be going on. Salmon and its fishy cousins offer many other vitamins and minerals that may help. Salmon has lots of selenium, for example, which is believed to fight tumors. One study found men who took selenium supplements had fewer cases of prostate cancer. Or perhaps just replacing red meat with fish does the trick.

▪ ▪ ▪ ▪ *Cook's corner* ▪ ▪ ▪ ▪

Love salmon? Here are a few things you may not know about this popular fish.

- Lox is a form of thinly sliced salmon that's been smoked. Some people enjoy it with cream cheese on a bagel. But lox has loads of sodium, so it may not fit into your diet if you're watching your salt.

- You may find something called "red caviar" at the grocery store. It's salmon eggs or roe, considered a delicacy by some. But it is not actual caviar, which by definition is roe from sturgeon.

- The flesh of wild salmon is naturally pink. Farm-raised salmon should have gray flesh since they don't eat the same food as their wild cousins. But people expect salmon to be pink, so farmers add dye to salmon food to change the fish's color.

Sardines

Pop open a can packed with nutrition

Ever heard of something being "packed like sardines"? That's because these tasty treats often come lined up shoulder to shoulder in small cans. In fact, "sardines" is the name of a children's game that involves crowding players into tight spaces. If you want a lot of nutrition packed into a tiny package, sardines are the way to go.

Sardines are a picnic favorite because they're easy to store and carry, and they're ready to eat right out of the can. Sardines in cans actually may be small herrings or similar fish, but they're all in the same family. One can of sardines gives

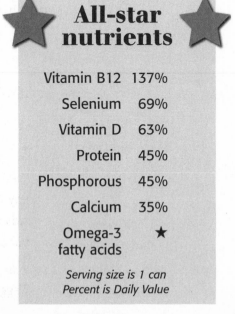

All-star nutrients

Vitamin B12	137%
Selenium	69%
Vitamin D	63%
Protein	45%
Phosphorous	45%
Calcium	35%
Omega-3 fatty acids	★

Serving size is 1 can
Percent is Daily Value

you a robust serving of vitamins B12 and D, along with minerals like selenium, phosphorous, and calcium. They're also supercharged with a hefty portion of protein and a good helping of healthy omega-3 fatty acids. As fatty fish go, they're relatively safe from contaminants. This tried-and-true convenience food makes a truly fine kettle of fish.

■ ■ ■ ■ ■ **Boost the benefits** ■ ■ ■ ■ ■

Canned sardines come in many flavors and varieties — packed in oil or water, flavored with mustard sauce or hot chili peppers, with or without salt. Your choice may depend on price, taste, and your health needs.

Pick sardines canned in water or tomato sauce if you're watching your weight. They're lower in calories than those in oil. And don't think you're getting the benefits of extra omega-3 fatty acids from oil-packed sardines. Many use soybean or olive oil rather than fish oil. Finally, if you're on a low-sodium diet, check the label for sardines with no salt added.

Crunch osteoporosis with bone-building fish. Pick canned sardines with the bones included, and you'll get a double dose of bone protection. Osteoporosis, the gradual loss of bone mass and strength as you age, can be slowed or prevented by getting more calcium and vitamin D in your diet.

Dairy products like milk and yogurt are the favorite sources of calcium and vitamin D for many people. But marine calcium — powdered fish bones or cartilage — is another great source. Researchers compared marine calcium with calcium from milk to see which your body absorbs better. They found that marine calcium is just as good as dairy calcium.

Don't fret if you're not thrilled with the thought of eating powdered fish bones. You can get the same benefit from the real thing. A can of sardines with bones gives you more than one-third the calcium and nearly two-thirds the vitamin D you need every day. Without bones, the calcium content in sardines can drop to 10 percent or less.

■ ■ ■ ■ *Cook's corner* ■ ■ ■ ■

Fresh sardines are not easy to find because they spoil quickly. If you get lucky and find some, grill or broil the fish without adding too much fat. You can also buy them salted, smoked, or canned. Sardines last about two days fresh and six months frozen. Canned sardines can last a year or more at 65 degrees Fahrenheit or lower. Turn the cans over occasionally to keep the fish moist.

Shrimp

Tiny crustacean delivers jumbo nutrition

Forrest Gump's army buddy was right when he said, "Shrimp is the fruit of the sea." Shrimp comes in a range of different types, living in both salt and fresh water. The shrimp on your dinner plate may have been harvested from the sea or grown in a fishery. Not only is it tasty and full of nutrition, it can be made into many dishes — from gumbo to sandwiches and everything in between.

■■■■■ Boost the benefits ■■■■■

Shrimp don't have much fat, but they do carry a lot of cholesterol. One 3-ounce serving has 166 milligrams. That's more than half of what you should have in a day.

A new type of shrimp could let you enjoy your favorite shrimp dishes while you watch your cholesterol. EcoFish has developed an all-natural white shrimp that has 30 percent less cholesterol than traditional shrimp. It's available frozen, both cooked and uncooked. Look for EcoFish in the frozen seafood section at your grocery store.

Many people think of shrimp as a special treat, but it's also good for you. Shrimp is low in fat, high in protein, and carries an impressive set of nutrients. You can count on getting important minerals like selenium and iron, along with vitamins like vitamin E and vitamin B12. Shrimp gets its pretty pink color from astaxanthin, an antioxidant in the same family as beta carotene. It's also a source of healthy omega-3 fatty acids, although shrimp doesn't have as much as fish like salmon and trout.

Some people are allergic to shrimp and other shellfish. Others need to watch their cholesterol, which is fairly high in shrimp. But if you don't have those problems, feel free to visit the shrimp buffet as often as possible.

Easy way to power up your muscles. It's common for your

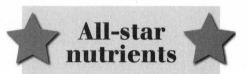

All-star nutrients

Selenium	48%
Protein	36%
Vitamin B12	21%
Iron	15%
Vitamin E	6%
Astaxanthin	★
Omega-3 fatty acids	★

Serving size is 3 ounces, cooked
Percent is Daily Value

muscles to become weaker as you get older. That's partly because you use them less for heavy lifting and other hard work. It could also be that you don't get enough of the important mineral selenium in your diet. Eating shrimp is an easy and delicious way to help solve that problem.

Selenium helps you make certain enzymes, natural chemicals that help your body function. One of these enzymes, called selenoprotein W, is believed to help muscles do their job. Research on nearly 900 older men and women in Italy found a connection between selenium in their blood and muscle strength. People with the least selenium also had the lowest scores for hand grip and knee and hip strength.

A small, 3-ounce serving of shrimp has nearly half the selenium you need in a day. Shrimp is also a good source of astaxanthin, a natural antioxidant believed to protect muscles from damage after strenuous exercise. Shrimp's vitamin E, which boosts muscle endurance, makes it a triple threat to muscle weakness.

▪ ▪ ▪ ▪ *Cook's corner* ▪ ▪ ▪ ▪

It takes a lot of work to prepare fresh shrimp. You have to wash the little critters, remove the tails and intestines, and take off the shells. If that's more trouble than you'd like, buy canned or frozen shrimp instead. Much of the shrimp sold as "fresh" actually has been frozen at some point anyway.

One pound of whole, raw shrimp will shrink to 8 ounces of cooked meat. That's because it loses about 25 percent of its weight in cleaning and another 25 percent in the cooking process.

Seafood allergies affect all ages

Shellfish — crab, lobster, shrimp, and crayfish — top the list of the most common food allergies. Children can outgrow allergies to milk or eggs. But just the opposite may be true for seafood and nut allergies. They can spring up in adults who've never had to deal with allergies.

Experts think your body may get confused by a new food or other substance, treating it like something you've had reactions to. In other cases, people move to a new part of the country and are exposed to new plants or other allergens — substances that cause reactions.

Allergic reactions to seafood or other foods can be serious, possibly including anaphylactic shock. You may have a skin reaction, swelling, intestinal or heart problems, breathing trouble, and even sudden death.

Don't take food allergies lightly. Take these precautions if you have a severe allergy to seafood or other triggers.

- Tell your family and friends about your allergy and how to help if you have a reaction.

- If your doctor has prescribed self-injectable epinephrine like EpiPen or Twinject, always carry it with you.

- Practice using your epinephrine, and teach family and friends how to use it.

- Carry an antihistamine like Benadryl. These are sometimes used along with epinephrine.

- Wear a medical bracelet or necklace with information about your allergy.

- Call 911 or go to a hospital if you have a reaction. Don't drive yourself there.

Trout

■ ■ ■ ■ ■ ■ ■ ■ ■

Fly fishers' favorite offers healthy fillets

You may think trout live in clear streams and lakes, but the one on your plate likely was raised on a farm. Trout was the first fish to be farm-raised to prevent its extinction. Some types of trout live in the ocean as adults and return upstream to spawn — just like their salmon cousin.

Also like salmon, steelhead trout and rainbow trout are good sources of omega-3 fatty acids. Trout gives you protein, vitamins like niacin and vitamin B12, and minerals including phosphorous and selenium.

The health benefits of trout may extend beyond eating it to catching it. In fact, a nonprofit group called Casting for Recovery offers fly-fishing retreats for women who have had breast cancer. The activity lets survivors enjoy nature, meet other women, and perform gentle exercise through fly fishing. Oh, and eating the tasty and healthy catch is a great bonus for anyone.

Cut your risk of memory failure in half. Eating fatty fish like steelhead trout or rainbow trout may help more than your heart. It may also protect your brain from age-related memory loss.

Your brain cells need DHA, one of the omega-3 fatty acids in fish. Experts think there may be a connection between loss of DHA and Alzheimer's disease. Researchers checked to see if people who eat more fish keep

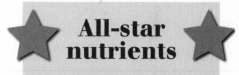

All-star nutrients

Vitamin B12	59%
Protein	34%
Niacin	31%
Phosphorous	19%
Selenium	15%
Omega-3 fatty acids	★

Serving size is 1 fillet
Percent is Daily Value

their memories sharper as they age. One study followed nearly 900 older men and women for an average of nine years, recording DHA levels in their blood and how sharp their minds stayed. Both Alzheimer's disease and other age-related dementia were recorded. People who ate the most fish had about half the risk of dementia as those who ate the least fish. Those who ate fish about three times a week did much better than those who ate it once a week.

■ ■ ■ ■ ■ **Boost the benefits** ■ ■ ■ ■ ■

Trout is quick and easy to prepare. It has tiny scales and thin skin that don't need to be removed. Trout traditionally is served fried, but try another method for a healthier option. It can be broiled, grilled, poached, baked, or steamed for a meal with less added fat.

Another study looked at more than 200 older men in the Netherlands for five years. It found that men who regularly ate fish were more likely to maintain a sharp mind than men who did not eat fish. The study concluded that one serving of fatty fish a week was enough to lessen memory loss.

Keep your eyesight sharper — for longer. It's common to feel that your eyes are weakening as you get older. People who suffer from retinitis pigmentosa (RP) know their eyes truly are weaker. This hereditary condition first makes it difficult to see at night, then harms your side vision, and finally may cause blindness.

Eating trout — or other oily fish like salmon, tuna, or sardines — may help slow down vision loss in people with RP. Trout has lots of the omega-3 fatty acid DHA, which certain cells in your eyes need to work right. These photoreceptor cells capture light, turn it into pictures, and send them to your brain. Studies show people with RP who ate fatty fish twice a week kept their vision longer than people who didn't. That could mean more years of seeing well enough to read, drive, and enjoy your favorite hobby.

Add a side of asparagus to your trout dinner for double protection. Asparagus serves up a hefty portion of vitamin A, also believed to slow vision loss in RP. And both DHA and vitamin A may ward off other causes of vision loss, like macular degeneration.

▪▪▪▪ *Cook's corner* ▪▪▪▪

Trout has a delicate flavor that is easily overwhelmed. Keep your cooking method simple so you can appreciate its natural taste. Trout — like other fish and meats — must be fully cooked to kill any bacteria that could make you sick. Don't trust your eyes that the trout is done. Instead, use a meat thermometer to be sure the temperature inside the fish reaches 145 degrees Fahrenheit. An instant-read meat thermometer gives you the correct temperature in seconds.

Balance cancer protection with tuna safety

You may be able to cut your risk of cancer by eating tuna or other fatty fish. Experts think the omega-3 fatty acids in fish may block natural body chemicals that help tumor cells grow.

Researchers followed about 48,000 men for 12 years, recording how much fish they ate and how many developed prostate cancer. The men who ate fatty fish more than three times a week had less risk of prostate cancer. Eating shellfish or taking fish oil supplements didn't seem to help. In another study, men in Sweden who ate fatty fish at least once a week had fewer cases of prostate cancer than those who never ate fish.

Tuna and some other fish also have lots of selenium. This important mineral is believed to fight tumors.

But don't go hog wild over canned tuna. Tests by the U.S. Food and Drug Administration have confirmed some may be contaminated with mercury. Follow these rules to stay safe.

- **Read the label.** Experts agree most chunk light tuna is less likely to be contaminated with mercury than solid light tuna. Both are safer than albacore tuna, which comes from larger fish.

- **Avoid damage to developing bodies.** Women of childbearing age or who are pregnant or nursing may want to avoid canned tuna and choose other types of fish. The same goes for children who weigh less than 45 pounds.

- **Enjoy tuna within limits.** Men and older women may safely eat up to three cans of chunk light tuna per week. If you prefer solid light or albacore tuna, limit it to one can a week.

Punch up your diet with low-fat dairy

Eggs

Crack open a wealth of good health

Eggs have gotten a bad rap lately, most of it undeserved. They're inexpensive, easy to fix, and chock-full of nutrients. For starters, they're an excellent source of complete, high-quality, easy-to-digest protein as well as the B vitamins biotin, riboflavin, and B12; the mineral selenium; the essential nutrient choline; and lutein and zeaxanthin, two phyto-chemicals crucial to your vision.

They are high in cholesterol, but don't let this scare you. Eggs don't appear to boost heart disease risk. Cholesterol in food does not cause a rise in blood cholesterol in 70 percent of people. Those who are cholesterol-sensitive, the other 30 percent, see a rise in both HDL and LDL levels. What's more, their large-particle LDL, the safer kind, rises. Their small-particle LDL, the type linked to heart disease, does not.

That doesn't mean you can eat a three-egg omelet every morning. Enjoying them occasionally won't hurt most people and may actually help you get the nutrients you need as you get older.

Protect your peepers from AMD. Age-related macular degeneration (AMD) is the leading cause of blindness in people over age 60. It attacks your eye's macula, the part you use for sharp, central vision. Fortunately, what you eat can make a big difference in whether you get it.

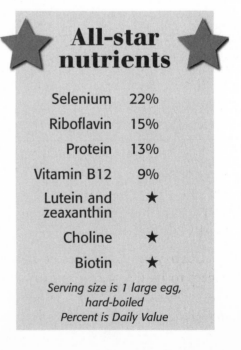

All-star nutrients

Selenium	22%
Riboflavin	15%
Protein	13%
Vitamin B12	9%
Lutein and zeaxanthin	★
Choline	★
Biotin	★

Serving size is 1 large egg, hard-boiled
Percent is Daily Value

310

▪ ▪ ▪ ▪ ▪ Boost the benefits ▪ ▪ ▪ ▪ ▪

An egg is an egg — or it used to be. Now you can buy them enriched with all sorts of nutrients, including omega-3, lutein, and vitamin E. These special eggs cost more, and if you eat a balanced diet, you probably don't need the added nutrients. However, they won't hurt if you feel better about eating them.

Pasteurized eggs, on the other hand, add another layer of protection against salmonella poisoning. The pasteurization process claims to kill nearly 100 percent of salmonella inside the eggshell. Keep in mind, your risk of getting sick is low to begin with, but if you are elderly or have a weakened immune system, pasteurized eggs may be worth the extra cost.

One sure-fire way to get healthier eggs — cook up an omelet with good-for-you vegetables, mushrooms, low-fat shredded cheese, or salsa.

Two plant carotenoids, lutein and zeaxanthin, seem to lower your risk of AMD by protecting your lenses and absorbing the damaging ultraviolet (UV) light that enters your eyes. Luckily, egg yolks are excellent sources of both lutein and zeaxanthin, and the lutein in eggs is three times more absorbable than lutein from spinach.

Studies show eating foods rich in these two carotenoids can boost levels inside the macula. Sure enough, elderly people who ate one egg daily for five weeks raised their lutein levels 26 percent and zeaxanthin 38 percent. Even better, eating a daily egg did not meaningfully raise their cholesterol.

Curb your liver cancer risk. Eggs may be the last food you'd expect to battle cancer, but eating eggs lowered people's risk of liver cancer nearly 70 percent in one study. Three cancer-fighting nutrients in eggs may have something to do with it.

- In rat studies, choline shortages triggered the development of liver cancer and made rats more vulnerable to cancer-causing compounds. In people, a deficiency leads to fatty livers because choline helps move triglycerides out of your liver.

- Low levels of selenium are linked to higher rates of liver cancer, especially in people with hepatitis B or C. Experts suspect this mineral also boosts your immune system, helps keep tumors from growing, and affects how your body processes cancer-causing compounds.

- Too little vitamin B12 in your diet keeps your body from absorbing folate from food. A folate shortage, in turn, results in weaker strands of DNA inside your cells. Weak DNA is more prone to damage, and DNA damage is a major risk factor for cancer.

Unique cure for brittle nails. What's good for a horse could be good for humans, too. The B-vitamin biotin effectively treats hoof problems in horses, and several studies show it may strengthen brittle nails. In one, women who got more biotin noticed less splitting, and fingernails become 25 percent thicker. Next to liver, eggs are one of the best food sources of biotin. Milk, fish, nuts, and whole-grain cereals also pack a healthy dose.

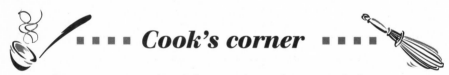

▪ ▪ ▪ ▪ *Cook's corner* ▪ ▪ ▪ ▪

Store eggs pointed-end down to keep the air inside from displacing the yolk, but don't keep them on the refrigerator door — they won't stay cool enough. Also, avoid washing eggs before storing. This strips away the shell's protective coating, making it easier for germs to sneak inside. Wipe dirty eggshells with a dry cloth, instead.

You'll find it easier to peel boiled eggs if you add two tablespoons of vinegar to the cooking water. Rinse hard-boiled eggs immediately under cold water to keep the grayish-green ring from forming around the yolk.

Make smart cheese choices

From feisty feta to low-key mozzarella, cheeses come in every available taste, texture, and variety. Their nutritional content can differ just as much as their flavor or color, especially if you choose low- or reduced-fat cheeses. See how your favorite slices stack up in calories, fat, and several important nutrients.

Cheese (1 ounce)	Cal.	Sat. fat (g)	Calcium (mg)	Sodium (mg)	Protein (g)	B12 (mcg)
Cheddar (low-fat)	113 (48)	6 (1)	202 (116)	174 (171)	7.0 (6.8)	0.2 (0.1)
Cottage cheese (1%)	29 (20)	1 (0)	16.8 (17.1)	113 (114)	3.5 (3.5)	0.2 (0.2)
Cream cheese (low-fat)	98 (65)	6 (3)	22.4 (31.4)	82.9 (82.9)	2.1 (3.0)	0.1 (0.2)
Feta	74	4	138	312	4.0	0.5
Monterey (low-fat)	104 (88)	5 (4)	209 (197)	150 (158)	6.9 (7.9)	0.2 (0.2)
Mozzarella (part-skim)	84 (71)	4 (3)	141 (219)	176 (173)	6.2 (6.8)	0.6 (0.2)
Parmesan	121	5	311	428	10.8	0.6
Provolone (reduced fat)	98 (77)	5 (3)	212 (212)	245 (245)	7.2 (6.9)	0.4 (0.4)
Ricotta (part-skim)	48 (39)	2 (1)	58 (76.2)	23.5 (35)	3.2 (3.2)	0.1 (0.1)
Swiss (low-fat)	106 (50)	5 (1)	221 (269)	54 (73)	7.5 (8.0)	0.9 (0.5)
Velveeta (low-fat)	85 (62)	4 (2)	130 (161)	420 (444)	4.6 (5.5)	~ (~)

Source: NutritionData.com

Milk

■ ■ ■ ■ ■ ■

Grab a cold glass of goodness

Humans have certainly learned to make the most of milk. These days, most milk comes from cows, but you can also get it from goats, sheep, donkeys, horses, buffaloes, and even reindeer.

Good thing. It supplies many of the key nutrients you need to live. Milk packs complete, high-quality protein, a variety of B vitamins including B12, and the minerals calcium, magnesium, phosphorus, zinc, iodine, and selenium. In the United States, vitamin D is added to store-bought milk to help you absorb and use calcium. Low-fat and skim milk may also be fortified with vitamin A. Lactose, a sugar found only in milk, helps you absorb calcium and phosphorus, and it may promote the growth of friendly bacteria in your digestive tract.

That's just the beginning. From your heart to your bones, milk has the nutrients to help your body stay strong.

Simple way to build strength and lose fat. Gulping a glass of skim milk after exercising can help you build more muscle and keep what you already have. Men drank a glass of fat-free milk immediately after working out with weights, then another glass one hour later. They built more muscle and lost more fat than men drinking high-protein soy drink or a high-carbohydrate beverage.

Your body seems to absorb and put to use more of the

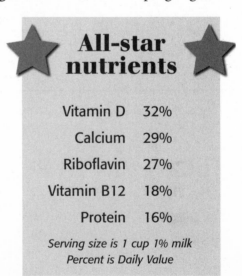

All-star nutrients

Vitamin D	32%
Calcium	29%
Riboflavin	27%
Vitamin B12	18%
Protein	16%

Serving size is 1 cup 1% milk
Percent is Daily Value

protein in milk. Timing matters, too. Getting protein immediately after exercising maximizes the amount of muscle you build.

Lower the boom on high blood pressure. Eat more dairy, particularly milk, to lower your blood pressure. Drinking milk may make a difference, particularly if you are salt-sensitive.

- One study found that Dutch seniors who ate the most dairy products tended to have lower blood pressure. Researchers say getting more daily dairy could help people with or at risk of high blood pressure.

- A Harvard study confirms that eating more dairy foods, particularly milk, may lower your blood pressure. In this study, the more dairy that people ate, the lower their blood pressure. The biggest drop came from eating lots of dairy but limiting saturated fat to less than 11 percent of their daily calories.

Milk's calcium and a special type of fat called alpha-linolenic acid (ALA) may keep blood pressure low. This delicious drink also gives you potassium and magnesium, known for battling high blood pressure. Plus, it's rich in vitamin B12, a nutrient that may help prevent cardiovascular diseases.

Only low-fat, not high-fat, dairy does the trick. Saturated fat seems to cancel out some of milk's benefits, so choose low-fat (1%) or fat-free (skim) milk whenever possible.

Employ triple threat against cancer. Develop a taste for dairy products, especially milk, and you could slash your risk of certain cancers. For starters, two new studies link vitamin D and calcium to colon cancer protection. A Korean study found that getting plenty of calcium lowered people's risk 27 percent, while vitamin D lowered it up to 33 percent. In a Hawaiian study, men saw a 30-percent drop linked to calcium and a 28-percent drop linked to vitamin D, while women earned a 36-percent drop from calcium.

Getting more calcium from food cut the risk of breast cancer in half among 3,600 women, giving particular protection to premenopausal women. Other research in a group of 30,000 women linked both calcium and vitamin D from food to lower rates of breast cancer, but only in premenopausal women. In yet another study, milk and yogurt were linked to lower rates of liver cancer.

The vitamin B12 found in milk helps wage an anti-cancer campaign, too. This nutrient plays an important role in preventing cancer, particularly breast cancer. Your body needs B12 to free another vitamin, folate, from food. Your cells then use folate to build healthy DNA, your body's genetic "blueprint." Getting too little B12 leaves the folate trapped in food, unusable by your body. This folate shortage, in turn, causes your body to build weak DNA that is more susceptible to cancer-causing changes. So think of milk as a triple-threat against cancer, with its rich stores of calcium, vitamin D, and B12.

■ ■ ■ ■ ■ Boost the benefits ■ ■ ■ ■ ■

You can buy milk fortified with many nutrients. Consider these to make the most of this beverage.

- ■ vitamin D, a no-brainer for bone health

- ■ extra calcium beyond what naturally comes in milk, which studies show may help boost bone density

- ■ omega-3, folic acid, and oleic acid, the combination of which may battle high cholesterol, triglycerides, blood sugar, and homocysteine

You can reap all the benefits without the drawbacks by ditching whole and 2% milk for skim or 1% milk. The saturated fat found naturally in dairy foods contributes to heart disease, obesity, and some cancers. Skim, nonfat, and buttermilk contain the least fat, while 1% milk comes in a healthy second.

Bolster bones and prevent falls. Milk supplies lots of calcium, and calcium from food builds stronger bones than calcium from supplements. Fortified milk also gives you vitamin D. Recent research suggests that meeting your needs for D may actually be more important than calcium for bone density. New evidence shows milk proteins play a big role in building bones, too. That means milk may be better for bone strength than other dairy foods. That's especially important for women over age 50, who are at higher risk for brittle bones that break easily.

Milk's combination of calcium and vitamin D may help protect your bones in another way, too. A recent study found it reduced older women's risk of falling by 46 percent. Less active women benefited even more, with 65 percent less risk of falling. Experts explain that vitamin D deficiencies contribute to muscle weakness, a major risk factor in falls. Plus, your muscles lose the ability to use vitamin D with age. All this means you need more of it as you get older to keep your muscles working well.

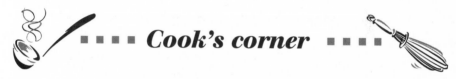

▪ ▪ ▪ ▪ *Cook's corner* ▪ ▪ ▪ ▪

- Lengthen milk's shelf life by refrigerating it at or below 40 degrees. Adding a pinch of salt or a teaspoon of baking soda to milk when it nears its expiration date can help you get a few more good days out of it. Never pour unused milk back into the container.

- If you prefer canned milk, just be sure to turn the can upside down every two months, and refrigerate in a solid-colored container after opening.

- Cooking with milk doesn't have to be hard. When heating it on the stove, spread a thin layer of unsalted butter on the bottom of the pan to keep the milk from sticking. There's no need to scald pasteurized milk in recipes because pasteurized milk has already been scalded.

Mozzarella cheese

■ ■ ■ ■ ■ ■ ■ ■ ■ ■ ■ ■ ■ ■ ■ ■ ■ ■

Say 'cheese' to beat disease

Talk about your aged cheeses — archeologists say cheese-making began as long as 10,000 years ago. The Romans were the real connoisseurs, exporting their love of it around the world. When the Roman Empire fell, church monasteries kept cheese-making knowledge alive during the Middle Ages. Now, you can enjoy more than 1,000 different varieties of cheese around the world, with over 350 of them from France alone.

Mozzarella is an unripened, stretched-curd cheese. It doesn't undergo the same aging and ripening process as varieties such as cheddar, Brie, or Muenster. Instead, the curd from milk is stored in water until it reaches the right rubbery consistency, then stretched and kneaded into shape.

Like most other dairy products, mozzarella is a great source of calcium for strong bones as well as protein and phosphorus. Learn how to love cooking with mozzarella and how it can love you back.

Put the brakes on high blood sugar. Good news for people with diabetes — you no longer have to cut all your favorite high-GI foods from your diet. Topping certain foods with cheese can drop the overall glycemic index of a meal to safer levels.

Potatoes are considered a "high" food on the glycemic index, while pasta is "medium" and toast is "low." Sprinkling about one cup of shredded

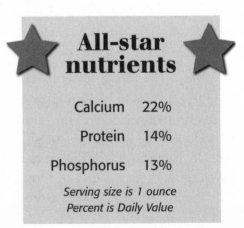

All-star nutrients

Calcium	22%
Protein	14%
Phosphorus	13%

Serving size is 1 ounce
Percent is Daily Value

cheddar cheese on each of these foods significantly lowered their GI value, dropping them all — even potatoes — into the "low" range.

■ ■ ■ ■ ■ **Boost the benefits** ■ ■ ■ ■ ■

Generally, it takes 11 pounds of milk to make just one pound of cheese. No wonder this treat can be such a concentrated source of saturated fat. But don't despair. It's easy to enjoy cheese and still cut back on fat.

■ Use low-fat or fat-free cheese to add flavor to salads instead of pouring on fatty dressings. Just a little strongly flavored, hard cheese like sapsago and Romano add lots of taste.

■ Save fresh mozzarella for special occasions, and use the part-skim or fat-free supermarket cheese for everyday cooking. Fresh mozzarella is usually made from whole-fat milk, so it contains much more saturated fat.

Researchers say adding a little fat to a meal lowers your glycemic response. That is, the fat in food makes your stomach empty more slowly into your small intestine. This, in turn, causes your body to absorb carbohydrates more slowly into your bloodstream, which leads to a lower, more gradual rise in blood sugar after eating. Since one of the biggest challenges in diabetes is managing blood sugar highs and lows, you may want to say "hooray" for cheese.

Delicious way to fight dry mouth. Eating cheese with beneficial bacteria added to it could make your mouth very happy. Elderly people who ate about half a cup of shredded cheese daily made with live, friendly bacteria called probiotics reduced the amount of Candida yeast growing in their mouths and lowered their risk of dry mouth. Those who ate just regular cheese, without these helpful bacteria, saw a rise in the amount of unfriendly yeast living in their mouths. Some companies now offer probiotic cheese along with their traditional cheeses. Try one and see if it whets your whistle.

Hidden migraine trigger

Migraine sufferers may want to avoid mozzarella. It contains tyramine, a compound that can trigger migraines in some people. Usually, the longer cheese ages, the more tyramine it contains. Mozzarella is the exception. Blue cheese, Brie, cheddar, feta, Gorgonzola, Muenster, Parmesan, and Swiss are also rich in this compound.

▪▪▪▪ *Cook's corner* ▪▪▪▪

- Low-fat cheese may be better for you, but it's notoriously hard to melt. One easy fix — soak slices in water or broth for two minutes, then melt as usual. They'll ooze just like full-fat cheese.

- You'll get more flavorful cheese if you let it warm to room temperature before serving. If grating, however, grate while cold. Pop it in the freezer for 10 minutes to chill, if necessary.

- Use mozzarella soon after buying. It goes bad faster than most, since it's a soft cheese with more moisture than other varieties.

Yogurt

■ ■ ■ ■ ■ ■ ■ ■ ■ ■

Creamy treat boosts whole-body health

One of the healthiest, most versatile dairy foods was probably discovered by accident 4,000 years ago when nomads stumbled upon a new way to preserve milk. Asia, the Middle East, and Mediterranean countries have enjoyed yogurt for years. Now it's finally catching on across the water in the United States.

Friendly bacteria, usually either *Streptococcus thermophilus* or *Lactobacillus bulgaricus*, are added to pasteurized milk, heated, then cooled. The bacteria turn some of the lactose, or dairy sugar, in yogurt into lactic acid, the secret to its tangy taste. The more types of bacteria, the tangier the yogurt.

This one creamy, delicious food fortifies the immune system, bolsters bones, helps you lose weight, prevents digestive disorders, and even fights bad breath, thanks to its amazing combination of calcium, protein, and friendly bacteria. Like milk, it's also an excellent source of phosphorus, potassium, and B vitamins. Discover this super food today.

Sweeten your breath with a creamy dessert. Banishing your bad breath may be as easy as eating half a cup of yogurt. Japanese researchers took 24 people with halitosis, or bad breath, and gave them about three and a half ounces of plain, sugarless yogurt every day.

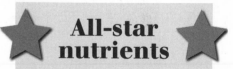

All-star nutrients

Calcium	45%
Phosphorus	35%
Riboflavin	31%
Protein	26%
Vitamin B12	23%
Beneficial bacteria	★

Serving size is 8 ounces, low fat
Percent is Daily Value

After six weeks, 80 percent of the yogurt-eaters experienced a drop in the smelly sulfur compound hydrogen sulfide, a major culprit behind bad breath. They also had fewer harmful bacteria on their tongues, less plaque, and healthier gums. The yogurt they ate contained live bacteria, so shop for sugar-free yogurt with "live and active cultures."

■ ■ ■ ■ ■ **Boost the benefits** ■ ■ ■ ■ ■

Shop for yogurt with the latest expiration date, and be sure to buy the low-fat and fat-free varieties to reap all the benefits without the saturated fat. Watch out, too, for flavored yogurt made with loads of added sugar. Instead, buy plain yogurt, and add your own honey or fruit for natural sweetness.

Look for labels that say "live," "active," or "viable" cultures. This means the yogurt contains living bacteria, the only kind that benefits your digestive system. You can cook with yogurt, but heat will kill these good bugs.

Ditch the discomfort of diarrhea. If diarrhea has you down, maybe you should eat more yogurt. Eating yogurt regularly can help treat diarrhea caused by stomach bugs and may prevent the kind caused by antibiotics.

A review of medical research in children showed *Lactobacillus*, a good bacteria in yogurt, relieved diarrhea from bacterial infections. Antibiotics, on the other hand, trigger diarrhea by upsetting the balance of good to bad bacteria in your gut, leading to an overgrowth of the bad bugs. In another review, eating yogurt made with friendly *Lactobacilli* or *Bifidobacteria* helped prevent bouts of antibiotic-induced diarrhea in two out of four studies, leading researchers to conclude that probiotics may provide some benefit. Again, look for yogurt with "live and active" bacterial cultures to try this remedy.

Immunize yourself against infections. Believe it or not, the bacteria naturally found in your gut play a big role in keeping your immune system healthy. Yogurt can help maintain the balance of gut bugs, giving you stronger immunity against infections like pneumonia.

Cutting all fermented foods out of your diet actually suppresses your immune system, but research shows eating yogurt can bring it back to normal. Experts think yogurt containing live bacteria can strengthen your immune system and help it fight off infections. In a group of elderly people, those who ate yogurt made with the bacterium *Lactobacillus casei* recovered from illnesses 20 percent faster. In animals, yogurt helps their immune systems recover from nutritional deficiencies, regain their normal immune strength, and fight off respiratory infections such as pneumonia.

Sound strange? Your body has immune cells that make an illness-fighting compound called immunoglobulin. These amazing results make sense when you realize 80 percent of these cells live in your small intestine. Eating yogurt with live bacteria triggers your body to make more of these immune cells and prompts them to make more immunoglobulin. Plus, yogurt stimulates other immune cells, called T-cells, to make infection-fighting substances called cytokines.

Win at weight loss with calcium-filled treat. It's not a magic pill, but adding this creamy and delicious treat to your diet may help you shed more pounds and burn fat faster than cutting calories alone.

Scientists say the calcium in yogurt may keep your body from absorbing the fat in foods. What's more, calcium in food seems to help you lose more weight and fat than calcium in supplements. One group of overweight dieters lost 61 percent more body fat and 22 percent more pounds just by trimming their calories and eating six ounces of yogurt three times a day.

Yogurt makes a great between-meal snack. Both thick, spoonable yogurt and a liquid yogurt drink will leave you feeling fuller and more satisfied than fruit juice or other dairy drinks. It may not help you eat less at your next meal, but it could tide you over better between meals and help you cut back on less-healthy snacks.

Plus, building yogurt into your weight-loss plan will give you the calcium you need to keep your bones strong. Women tend to lose bone density while losing weight, perhaps because they cut back on dairy products in an effort to cut calories. Unfortunately, cutting calories also seems to limit the amount of calcium you absorb.

The solution — make low-fat and fat-free yogurt part of your diet plan. Women who got between 1,000 and 1,800 mg of calcium daily while dieting did not lose bone mass, compared to other weight-watchers. Eight ounces of low-fat yogurt provides you with 448 mg of calcium, almost half the low end of what you need.

▪ ▪ ▪ ▪ *Cook's corner* ▪ ▪ ▪ ▪

Yogurt makes almost any dish even better. Dip fruits and vegetables in flavored yogurt, like vanilla, add it to stroganoff or guacamole, or use it to top baked potatoes and cold cereals. Plus, it makes a great base for smoothies — a healthier alternative to milk shakes. Substitute plain, low- or fat-free yogurt in place of mayonnaise, heavy cream, or sour cream in recipes, or enjoy yogurt as a snack unto itself by stirring in honey, fruit, or granola.

Yogurt curdles easily when cooked. You can cut down on curdling by letting it warm up to room temperature before slowly heating it. If substituting it for cream in a hot dish, stir a little cornstarch into the yogurt to keep it from separating. Add one teaspoon of cornstarch for every cup of yogurt.

Quick guide: nutrition by condition

Aging skin

■ ■ ■ ■ ■ ■ ■ ■ ■ ■ ■ ■ ■ ■ ■

In case you hadn't noticed, your skin changes with age, developing what some might call "character" — otherwise known as wrinkles, age spots, and dryness. It also becomes thinner and loses fat, making it less plump and smooth, and may take longer to heal.

Sunlight is one of the biggest culprits behind skin aging. When the sun's rays hit your skin, they start a chemical reaction that creates free radicals. These unstable molecules damage skin cells, and over time the damage shows up as age-related wear and tear. It can also lead to skin cancer.

Fortunately, it's never to late to start protecting yourself. Stay out of the sun when it is strongest, use sunscreen with a sun protection factor (SPF) of 15 or higher, wear protective clothing, and avoid sunlamps and tanning beds at all costs. Many products claim to revitalize aging skin or reduce wrinkles, but the Food and Drug Administration has approved only a few for sun-damaged or aging skin. Various treatments soothe dry skin and reduce the appearance of age spots.

Some studies hint that a lifelong diet may affect how your skin ages. People who ate lots of fruits, vegetables, legumes, eggs, whole grains, nuts, water, and tea in one study showed less sun damage than people who ate mostly red meat, whole milk, butter, potatoes, and sugar. Begin babying your skin with these nutrients.

Nutrient	What it does	Food source
monounsaturated fatty acids (MUFAs)	reduce free-radical sun damage through anti-oxidant properties	olive oil almonds avocados
vitamin C	reduces free-radical sun damage through anti-oxidant properties	peppers broccoli artichokes
vitamin E	reduces free-radical sun damage through anti-oxidant properties	almonds, kiwi, spinach, sunflower seeds
water	plumps up skin cells to reduce appearance of lines	

Alzheimer's disease

■ ■ ■ ■ ■ ■ ■ ■ ■ ■ ■ ■ ■ ■ ■ ■ ■ ■ ■ ■

Alzheimer's disease (AD) is a brain disorder that usually begins after age 60. It leads to a severe loss of mental ability that interferes with your daily activities.

AD begins slowly. If you have AD, it first affects the parts of your brain that control thought, memory, and language. That means you may have trouble remembering things that happened recently or names of people you know. As time passes, symptoms get worse. You may not recognize family members, or you may have trouble speaking, reading, or writing. You may even forget how to brush your teeth or comb your hair. In the late stages of AD, people may become anxious or aggressive, or they may wander away from home. Eventually, they need total care.

Although none of the current treatments or drugs can stop Alzheimer's, some drugs may help keep symptoms from getting worse for a while. Researchers continue to seek ways to cure or prevent Alzheimer's disease. One study found that taking a traditional Chinese herb, ba wei di huang wan (BDW), can help reduce dementia symptoms and may even improve mood. Meanwhile, you can take nutritional steps that may help.

Nutrient	What it does	Food source
folate	helps the body make certain amino acids, building blocks of proteins	avocados honeydew melon black beans spinach
omega-3 fatty acids	reduce inflammation in brain's blood vessels	salmon tuna flaxseed
thiamin	needed for nerve signals to move from brain to other body parts	broccoli sunflower seeds beans asparagus
vitamin B12	helps produce neurotransmitters to carry nerve signals	crab salmon tuna dairy products

Asthma

■ ■ ■ ■ ■ ■ ■ ■ ■ ■ ■

When you have asthma, simply breathing can be a struggle. This chronic disease affects your airways, the tubes that carry air in and out of your lungs. The inside walls of your airways become sore and swollen, making them sensitive. These sensitive airways may react strongly to things you are allergic to or find irritating, such as cigarette smoke, cold air, dust, and mold. Exercise and certain foods, like eggs, peanuts, milk, wheat, soy, and citrus fruits, can also trigger a reaction.

And when your airways react, watch out. They narrow, so your lungs get less air. This can lead to wheezing, coughing, tightness in your chest, and trouble breathing, especially early in the morning or at night. An asthma attack happens when symptoms become worse than usual. In a severe asthma attack, your airways can close so much that your vital organs do not get enough oxygen. It can even kill you.

Drugs, usually taken through inhalers, can help treat asthma flare-ups and keep asthma symptoms under control. Luckily, nutrients found in common foods can also help you breathe easier.

Nutrient	What it does	Food source
beta carotene	improves lung capacity	carrots spinach
caffeine	relaxes bronchial tubes so airways remain open	coffee black and green tea colas chocolate
lycopene	with vitamin E, has antioxidant effect to prevent exercise-induced asthma attacks	tomatoes tomato juice watermelon guava
quercetin	works as antioxidant to reduce inflammation in the lungs	apples cherries cranberries spring onions
vitamin C	acts as natural antihistamine, anti-inflammatory, and antioxidant	kiwi artichokes blueberries sweet peppers

Benign prostatic hyperplasia

■ ■

Benign prostatic hyperplasia (BPH) is a problem with the prostate gland. Only men have this gland. It sits below your bladder and around your urethra, the passage urine follows to leave your body.

When you're a young man, your prostate is about the size of a walnut. As you age, it slowly grows larger. If the prostate gets too large, it can cause urinary problems.

Benign prostatic hyperplasia (BPH) is very common in older men. The prostate is enlarged but has no cancer. Over time, an enlarged prostate may press against the urethra, making it hard to urinate. It may cause dribbling after you urinate or a need to urinate often, especially at night.

Several different kinds of prostate problems can cause these symptoms — including BPH, infection, or prostate cancer. But only a doctor can tell one from another. Your doctor will do a rectal exam to check for BPH. You may also need special X-rays or scans to check your urethra, prostate, and bladder.

Treatments for BPH include regular checks by your doctor; drugs, like alpha blockers and finasteride; and surgery. Here are some nutrients that may also help.

Nutrient	What it does	Food source
isoflavones	natural plant chemicals that block conversion of testosterone to DHT, which causes prostate cell growth	soy beans soy milk tofu
lignans	work like hormones to block conversion of testosterone to DHT, which causes prostate cell growth	flaxseed berries whole grains
selenium	slows growth of prostate cells	mushrooms tuna
zinc	may help shrink an enlarged prostate or reduce inflammation	amaranth leaves crab mushrooms

Breast cancer

■ ■ ■ ■ ■ ■ ■ ■ ■ ■ ■ ■ ■ ■ ■ ■ ■ ■ ■ ■

Breast cancer affects one in eight women during their lives. In fact, it kills more women in the United States than any cancer except lung cancer. No one knows for sure why some women get breast cancer, but experts believe these factors raise your risk.

- *Age.* Your chance of getting breast cancer rises as you get older.

- *Genetics.* Two genes, BRCA1 and BRCA2, greatly increase your risk. Women who have family members with breast or ovarian cancer may wish to be tested for these genes.

- *Menstruation.* Beginning periods before age 12 or going through menopause after age 55 makes you more likely to develop breast cancer.

Other risks include being overweight, using hormone-replacement therapy, taking birth-control pills, drinking alcohol, not having children or having your first child after age 35, and having dense breasts. Men can get breast cancer, but the number of cases is small.

Scientists are eagerly studying certain foods and nutrients for their potential to thwart this deadly disease. Here are a few promising candidates.

Nutrient	What it does	Food source
fiber	changes pre-menopausal hormone levels to reduce tumor growth	wheat bran whole-wheat bread
isothiocyanates	stimulate enzymes in the body to block tumor-causing steroid hormones	cabbage broccoli Brussels sprouts
omega-3 fatty acids	compete with omega-6 fatty acids for enzymes to block tumor growth and make cancer-fighting byproducts	salmon trout sardines light tuna flaxseed
phytoestrogens	work like human hormones to suppress tumor growth	soy beans soy milk tofu

Cataracts

■ ■ ■ ■ ■ ■ ■ ■ ■ ■ ■ ■ ■ ■ ■

Just as a dark, cloudy sky can mean trouble, so can the clouding of your eye's lens. That's what happens when you have cataracts, a condition very common in older people. In fact, by age 80, more than half of all people in the United States either have a cataract or have had cataract surgery.

Common symptoms of cataracts include:

- blurry vision
- colors that seem faded
- glare
- poor nighttime vision
- double vision
- frequent prescription changes in your eyewear

Cataracts usually develop slowly, with gradual changes to your vision. New glasses, brighter lighting, anti-glare sunglasses, or magnifying lenses can help at first. You may also need surgery, which involves removing the cloudy lens and replacing it with an artificial lens. If left untreated, cataracts can lead to blindness.

Wearing sunglasses and a hat with a brim to block ultraviolet sunlight may help delay cataracts. You can further protect your eyes by quitting smoking, limiting your alcohol, and eating more of these healthy nutrients.

Nutrient	What it does	Food source
antioxidants (lutein, vitamins A, C, E)	fight free-radical damage to the eyes from sunlight	kiwi cauliflower honeydew melon broccoli
B-complex vitamins (niacin, thiamin, riboflavin)	deficiencies are related to cataracts in the center of the eye's lens	spelt tuna nectarines whole-wheat bread
protein	deficiencies are related to cataracts in the center of the eye's lens	eggs cheese salmon shrimp

Colds and flu

■ ■

Sneezing, coughing, a scratchy throat, and a stuffy nose – yep, you have a cold. During the course of a year, people in the United States suffer one billion colds.

Touch a surface covered with cold germs, then touch your eyes or nose and — just like that — you can catch it. You can also inhale the germs. Those telltale symptoms start within two or three days and can last from two days to two weeks. Washing your hands and staying away from people with colds will help you avoid getting sick.

Flu symptoms are different. They come on suddenly and are worse than those of the common cold. They may include body or muscle aches, chills, cough, fever, headache, and sore throat.

Flu, or influenza, is a respiratory infection caused by a number of viruses. The viruses pass through the air and enter your body through your nose or mouth. The flu can be serious or even deadly for elderly people, newborn babies, and people with certain chronic illnesses.

Sometimes it's hard to tell whether you have a cold or the flu. Remember this — colds rarely cause a fever or headaches, while flu almost never causes an upset stomach. Now check out the following nutrients for natural ways to nix these illnesses.

Nutrient	What it does	Food source
allicin	acts as natural antibiotic to kill germs	garlic
selenium	boosts immunity to fight infections	mushrooms oatmeal crab
vitamin C	may shorten duration of cold symptoms	sweet peppers kiwi limes
water	prevents dehydration	
zinc	boosts immunity to prevent infection	crab wheat bran amaranth leaves

Colon cancer

■ ■

Cancer of the colon or rectum is also called colorectal cancer. Although it is the fourth most common cancer in the United States, colorectal cancer is often curable if you catch it early enough.

You are more likely to develop colorectal cancer if you are over age 50, and the risk increases with age. You are also more likely to get it if you have:

- polyps — growths inside the colon and rectum that may turn into cancer.
- a diet that is high in fat.
- a family history or personal history of colorectal cancer.
- ulcerative colitis or Crohn's disease.

Symptoms can include blood in the stool, narrower stools, a change in bowel habits, and general stomach discomfort. However, you may not develop symptoms right away, so screening is important. Everyone who is 50 or older should be screened regularly. Treatments include surgery, chemotherapy, and radiation.

Foods and nutrients like these may help you avoid colon cancer.

Nutrient	What it does	Food source
anthocyanins	block growth of cancer cells	blueberries cherries
calcium	binds with bile acids in the colon to prevent polyps from forming	milk Chinese cabbage broccoli
fiber	grabs cancer-causing agents in digestive system and carries them from the body	whole grains brown rice black beans broccoli
folate	prevents DNA damage to keep cells from becoming malignant	spinach asparagus cauliflower artichokes
lutein	works as antioxidant to block tumor formation	spinach tomatoes nectarines broccoli

Constipation

■ ■

Everyone has a bout of constipation now and then. Infrequent bowel movements — say, fewer than three a week — and difficulty passing stool are the telltale signs of constipation. In most cases, it lasts only a short time and is not serious. But constipation may be a side effect of medication or a symptom of a more serious condition. It also becomes more common with age.

Constipation may lead to other problems. Straining during bowel movements can cause hemorrhoids, and hard stools may cause anal fissures, or tears in the skin near the anus.

Laxatives may be a short-term solution, but you don't want to become dependent on them. With just a few simple lifestyle changes, you can prevent constipation.

- Eat more fruits, vegetables, and grains, which are high in fiber, like the ones listed below.
- Drink plenty of water and other liquids.
- Get enough exercise.
- Take time to have a bowel movement when you need to.

Do not feel as though you must have a bowel movement every day. The normal frequency of bowel movements varies from person to person and ranges from three times a day to three times a week. However, if you experience a sudden change in bowel habits, check with your doctor.

Nutrient	What it does	Food source
insoluble fiber	softens and adds bulk to stool to keep bowels moving	whole-grain cereal figs broccoli
soluble fiber	forms gel in bowels to speed up stool	oatmeal black beans avocados
water	keeps stool soft to prevent intestinal blockage	

Depression

■ ■ ■ ■ ■ ■ ■ ■ ■ ■ ■ ■ ■ ■ ■ ■ ■

Depression is more than just a feeling of being "down in the dumps" or "blue" for a few days. It is a serious medical illness that affects your brain.

If you are one of the more than 20 million people in the United States who have depression, the feelings do not go away. Instead, they stick around and interfere with your everyday life. Symptoms of depression can include loss of interest or pleasure in activities you used to enjoy, sadness, weight changes, trouble sleeping, oversleeping, energy loss, feelings of worthlessness, or thoughts of death or suicide.

Depression can run in families, but it is much more common in women than in men. But the good news is that effective treatments are available for depression, including antidepressants and talk therapy. Most people do best by using both. Here are some foods that may help as well.

Nutrient	What it does	Food source
caffeine	boosts mood	coffee tea
folate	needed to produce neurotransmitters, which carry nerve signals; helps depression drugs work better	lettuce asparagus artichokes cauliflower honeydew melon spinach
omega-3 fatty acids	help neurotransmitters carry messages between nerve cells; boost levels of serotonin to improve mood	salmon sardines trout tuna flaxseed
tryptophan	needed to produce serotonin, which boosts mood	spinach shrimp crab
vitamin B12	helps folate produce neurotransmitters	crab salmon

Diabetes

■ ■ ■ ■ ■ ■ ■ ■ ■ ■ ■ ■ ■

Diabetes is a disease in which your blood sugar (glucose) levels are too high. You get blood sugar from the foods you eat, but a hormone called insulin usually helps you turn blood sugar into energy for your cells.

However, with type 1 diabetes, your body does not make insulin. And, in the more common type 2 diabetes, your body does not use insulin well and eventually loses the ability to make insulin at all. Without enough insulin, your blood sugar stays in your blood.

Over time, too much sugar in your blood can damage your eyes, kidneys, and nerves. Diabetes can also cause heart disease, stroke, and even the need to remove a limb.

Symptoms of type 2 diabetes may include fatigue, thirst, weight loss, blurred vision, and frequent urination. But some people have no symptoms and must take a blood test to determine whether they have diabetes. Exercise, weight control, and sticking to your meal plan are important ways to control your diabetes. The following nutrients can help. You should also monitor your blood sugar level and take medicine if your doctor prescribes it.

Nutrient	What it does	Food source
biotin	helps digest fats and carbohydrates, regulates blood sugar	eggs milk peanut butter
chromium	helps insulin move glucose from your blood into cells	romaine lettuce milk mushrooms
fiber	slows conversion of carbohydrates to glucose to avoid blood sugar spikes	oatmeal brown rice whole-wheat bread black beans
magnesium	helps prevent insulin resistance	avocados wheat bran black beans
omega-3 fatty acids	prevent insulin resistance	salmon flaxseed

Diarrhea

■ ■ ■ ■ ■ ■ ■ ■ ■ ■ ■ ■ ■ ■ ■

If you have loose, watery stools more than three times in one day, you've probably got diarrhea. You may also have cramps, bloating, nausea, and an urgent need to have a bowel movement.

Diarrhea can be caused by many things, including bacteria, viruses, or parasites; medicines; food intolerances; and a small crowd of diseases that affect the stomach, small intestine, or colon. But sometimes, no cause can be found.

Although usually not harmful, diarrhea can become dangerous or signal a more serious problem. For example, severe diarrhea can lead to dehydration, a condition in which your body loses too much of the important fluids and electrolytes your cells need to work properly. Symptoms of dehydration include dizziness, dry lips and mouth, a faster heart rate, rapid breathing, confusion, dark urine, and sometimes thirst.

The nutrients and foods below can help with bouts of diarrhea. But if you have severe stomach pain, a fever of more than 101 degrees Fahrenheit, blood in your stools or vomit, diarrhea for more than three days, or symptoms of dehydration, call your doctor right away.

Nutrient	What it does	Food source
anthocyanosides	kill *E. coli* bacteria	dried blueberries dried bilberries
pectin	soluble fiber that absorbs excess water in intestines to make stool firmer	bananas apples grapefruit carrots
potassium	helps regulate balance of water and other electrolytes in cells and tissues	bananas avocados cherries cabbage
probiotic bacteria	live active cultures such as acidophilus restore proper bacterial balance in intestines	yogurt fermented milk
water	replaces fluids lost from diarrhea, prevents dehydration	

Diverticular disease

■ ■ ■ ■ ■ ■ ■ ■ ■ ■ ■ ■ ■ ■ ■ ■ ■ ■ ■ ■

When you strain from constipation, you put too much pressure on your intestines, which weakens the intestinal wall. Over time, the weak spots start to give, forming small pouches, or diverticula. This condition, called diverticulosis, becomes more common with age. About half of people between the ages of 60 and 80 have diverticulosis, as does almost everyone over the age of 80.

Once you have diverticula, they don't go away. Although they aren't usually dangerous, undigested food and bacteria can get trapped inside the pouches and harden, causing infection or inflammation. This condition, called diverticulitis, can lead to serious complications. Inflamed pouches may rupture, spreading the infection to other organs. Luckily, only 10 to 25 percent of people with diverticulosis ever develop diverticulitis.

Diverticulosis does not usually cause symptoms. In some cases, however, people experience bloating, constipation, and pain in the lower left abdomen. Diverticulitis, on the other hand, can cause fever, chills, vomiting, diarrhea, constipation, loss of appetite, and pain in the lower left abdomen.

The pouches may bleed in both diverticulosis and diverticulitis, leaving blood in your stool. If you find blood in your stool, see your doctor. Usually the bleeding stops on its own, but if it persists, you might need medical treatment.

Make sure you get enough of these two nutrients to help you avoid the complications of diverticular disease.

Nutrient	What it does	Food source
fiber	bulks up and softens stool, helps it pass easily through intestines	whole-wheat bread wheat bran figs cauliflower broccoli
water	softens stool to prevent blockage, helps fiber flush out food particles from intestinal pouches	

Fatigue

■ ■ ■ ■ ■ ■ ■ ■ ■ ■ ■

Everyone gets the urge to sleep sometime, but fatigue is more than that. Fatigue is a feeling of weariness, tiredness, or a lack of energy and motivation. You may also hear it called exhaustion.

Fatigue can be a normal and important response to physical exertion, emotional stress, boredom, or lack of sleep. However, it can also be a sign of a more serious psychological or physical problem. Common causes include:

- anemia
- sleep disorders
- ongoing pain
- an allergy
- an underactive thyroid
- use of alcohol or illegal drugs
- depression or grief

Fatigue may also be a side effect of a condition like mononucleosis, congestive heart failure, diabetes, eating disorders, or cancer. Getting enough of the nutrients listed below may help your body fight fatigue. If good nutrition, sleep, or a low-stress environment doesn't ease or cure your fatigue, see your doctor.

Nutrient	What it does	Food source
iodine	used by thyroid to produce thyroxin, needed for metabolism	iodized salt seafood milk carrots
iron	carries oxygen on red blood cells to tissues	leeks spinach quinoa
magnesium	needed for muscle function, assists in melatonin production in brain for sound sleep	avocados black beans spinach amaranth wheat bran

Gallstones

■ ■ ■ ■ ■ ■ ■ ■ ■ ■ ■ ■ ■ ■ ■ ■

Gallstones form from cholesterol or other ingredients in bile, a fat-digesting liquid you make in your liver and store in your gallbladder.

When you need bile to help break down the fats you eat, it travels to the intestines. If stones have formed in the bile, they can lodge in the ducts that carry bile from the liver to the small intestine. If you experience fever, yellow-tinted skin or eyes, or persistent pain in your upper abdomen, call your doctor. You may have an infection or other serious problem.

Gallstones are more likely when bile ingredients have time to stagnate and build up in your gallbladder. The two types of gallstones are cholesterol stones and pigment stones. Cholesterol stones are the most common type, but small dark pigment stones made of bilirubin can also form. Gallstones may be as small as a grain of sand or as large as a golf ball. The gallbladder can develop just one large stone, hundreds of tiny stones, or almost any combination.

Many gallstones cause no symptoms, but doctors can remove the gallbladder if diet and lifestyle changes fail to stop repeated cases of painful gallstones. These nutrients may help.

Nutrient	What it does	Food source
caffeine	prevents symptoms of gallstones	coffee tea chocolate
fiber	moves food through digestive tract quickly to lower bile acid production	whole-grain bread black beans oatmeal figs
vitamin C	breaks down cholesterol so it doesn't turn into gallstones	fennel bell peppers kiwi blueberries

Gout

■ ■ ■ ■ ■ ■ ■

Gout is a painful condition that occurs when your body deposits uric acid, a waste product, in your joints and soft tissues instead of flushing it out of your body. It crystallizes in your joints, triggering bouts of pain, inflammation, swelling, redness, and stiffness. If not treated, gout attacks can become chronic, crippling your joints and limiting movement.

In many people, gout first strikes in the big toe, a condition called podagra. But you can get it in other joints and tissues, too, including your fingers, wrists, elbows, knees, ankles, and the insteps and heels of your feet. Uric acid can even form lumps under the skin surrounding your joints and covering the rim of your ears, or it can collect in your kidneys and cause kidney stones.

It tends to run in families, and men seem more likely than women to develop it. High blood pressure, obesity, alcohol abuse, and insulin resistance all raise your risk for gout.

Gout is a disease that often goes along with a rich diet — one reason it has been called the "disease of kings." That makes it a condition you can control by choosing foods wisely. You'll need to cut down on fatty foods; eat more fruits, vegetables, and whole grains; avoid alcohol; and exercise regularly.

Nutrient	What it does	Food source
anthocyanins	stop body from forming prostaglandins, which cause inflammation	cherries dried cherries blueberries raspberries red grapes
dairy protein	controls uric acid level in blood	milk cheese yogurt
water	flushes uric acid from tissues	

Hay fever

■ ■ ■ ■ ■ ■ ■ ■ ■ ■ ■ ■ ■ ■ ■ ■

Hay fever, or an allergy to pollen, affects about 35 million Americans, making it one of the most common types of allergies. Trees, grasses, and weeds produce pollen and release this fine, powdery material into the air you breathe during the spring, summer, and fall. You may experience different symptoms at different times of the year. It depends on the kinds of plants that grow where you live and what allergies you have.

Symptoms of hay fever include sneezing, coughing, and runny or clogged nose. You may also have itchy eyes, nose, and throat and watery, red, or swollen eyes.

No one is sure what causes allergies, but you are more likely to develop hay fever if your parents have it. Your doctor can help you decide how to treat your hay fever. You can avoid the things that cause your symptoms, use drugs to treat your symptoms, or get allergy shots.

Some people believe in eating a spoonful of local honey every day. The idea is that you'll become accustomed to the pollen used to make the honey — the same pollen that causes a hay fever reaction. You should also fit these nutrients into your diet.

Nutrient	What it does	Food source
omega-3 fatty acids	reduce inflammation	flaxseed walnuts
quercetin	regulates membranes to control histamine production	cherries cranberries spring onions
vitamin C	keeps body from making too much histamine	kiwi sweet peppers honeydew melon
vitamin E	affects inflammation, protects cell membranes	sunflower seeds olive oil avocados

Heartburn

■ ■ ■ ■ ■ ■ ■ ■ ■ ■ ■ ■ ■ ■ ■ ■ ■ ■

Heartburn is a painful burning feeling in your chest or throat. You get heartburn when stomach acid and other digestive juices back up into your esophagus, the tube that carries food to your stomach.

Almost everyone has heartburn sometimes. But if you have heartburn more than twice a week, you may have gastroesophageal reflux disease (GERD). Here's what you need to know.

A little valve that sits just above your stomach is supposed to protect your esophagus. In fact, this lower esophageal sphincter (LES) normally stays tightly shut except when food needs to enter your stomach. But with GERD, the LES does not seal up tightly enough to hold the digestive juices in your stomach. This allows contents of your stomach to back up into the esophagus and irritate it. Doctors call this reflux.

Medications, certain foods, and alcohol can bring on heartburn. Eating foods high in fat, especially fried foods, can make heartburn worse, Coffee, tea, and whole milk can cause problems, too. Try to eat more of the nutritional foods listed below. Extra weight puts pressure on your stomach and the LES so you're more likely to get heartburn. That's why doctors suggest you lose weight.

Treating heartburn is important because over time reflux can damage the esophagus — sometimes badly enough to lead to cancer. Fortunately, lifestyle changes can help, and your doctor can give you advice and treatment. If your heartburn comes with other symptoms such as crushing chest pain, you may be having a heart attack. Get help immediately.

Nutrient	What it does	Food source
fiber	prevents constipation, which can make heartburn worse	whole-wheat bread figs nectarines wheat bran
omega-3 fatty acids	substitute for saturated fats, which can worsen symptoms	trout flaxseed walnuts salmon
water	flushes digestive acids out of esophagus	

High blood pressure

■ ■ ■ ■ ■ ■ ■ ■ ■ ■ ■ ■ ■ ■ ■ ■ ■ ■ ■

If you've ever tried to run water through a garden hose that's been hardened by age or gunked up with hard-water deposits, you know how hard it is to get a good water flow. Blood flow through your arteries works the same way. Stiff or blocked arteries can make your heart strain to push blood through all your blood vessels. The result is high blood pressure, which damages both your heart and your blood vessels.

A blood pressure reading can tell you whether you have high blood pressure. The reading uses two numbers, the systolic and diastolic pressures, written one above or before the other. A reading of:

- 120/80 or lower is normal.
- 140/90 or higher is high blood pressure.
- 120 and 139 for the top number, or between 80 and 89 for the bottom number, is prehypertension.

High blood pressure usually has no symptoms, but it can cause serious problems such as stroke, heart failure, heart attack, and kidney failure. You can control high blood pressure through healthy lifestyle habits and taking medicines. Make sure you include these nutrients in your diet as well.

Nutrient	What it does	Food source
calcium	helps remove sodium	milk, cheese
omega-3 fatty acids	expand blood vessels, keep blood from clumping	salmon, tuna sardines flaxseed oil
potassium	balances sodium, dilates blood vessels, prompts sympathetic nervous system	bananas, avocados beans cherries fennel
magnesium	relaxes blood vessels, balances potassium and sodium	whole-wheat cereal broccoli, amaranth black beans
vitamin C	keeps blood vessel walls flexible	avocados nectarines

High cholesterol

▪▪▪▪▪▪▪▪▪▪▪▪▪▪▪▪▪▪▪▪▪▪▪▪▪▪▪▪▪▪

Cholesterol is a waxy, fat-like substance in some foods. Your body needs some cholesterol to build cell walls and make hormones. But if you have too much in your blood, it can stick to the walls of your arteries as plaque, blocking your arteries. Molecules called lipoproteins carry cholesterol through your bloodstream. Low-density lipoprotein (LDL) is considered "bad" because it carries cholesterol to your artery walls, where it causes damage. High-density lipoprotein (HDL) is "good" because it whisks cholesterol to your liver, where it gets eliminated from your body.

Besides cholesterol, you have another type of "bad" fat in your blood called triglycerides. They can wreak havoc of their own, lowering HDL levels and leading to blood clots and inflammation. Cholesterol and triglycerides are measured in milligrams per deciliter of blood, or mg/dL. Your target numbers vary — the higher your risk for heart disease, the lower you want your LDL.

Total cholesterol. Less than 200 mg/dL is best. Between 200 and 239 is borderline, and over 240 is high.

LDL. Below 100 mg/dL is ideal. If you're at very high risk, you should aim even lower — 70 mg/dL. Anything over 160 is high, while levels above 190 are very high and require medication.

HDL. Above 40 mg/dL is desirable, while levels above 60 mg/dL are optimal.

Triglycerides. Below 150 mg/dL is normal, from 150 to 199 is borderline high, and from 200 to 499 is high. Over 500 is very high.

Age and family history affect your risk, and while you can't change those, you can take steps to battle other risk factors. Exercise regularly, lose weight, quit smoking, and eat foods with these nutrients.

Nutrient	What it does	Food source
beta glucan	slows digestion, allows HDL to remove cholesterol	oatmeal, oat bran barley
lignans	lower cholesterol levels	flaxseed
lutein	keeps plaque from forming in arteries	kiwi, broccoli spinach
phytosterols	keep cholesterol from being absorbed in intestines	pistachios, sunflower seeds, amaranth

Insomnia

■ ■ ■ ■ ■ ■ ■ ■ ■ ■ ■ ■ ■ ■ ■ ■

Some people with insomnia may fall asleep easily enough but wake up too soon. Others simply can't fall asleep, or they have trouble both falling asleep and staying asleep. The result is low-quality sleep that doesn't make you feel refreshed when you wake up. Often, your insomnia is a symptom or a side effect of some other problem like one of these.

- illnesses, such as heart or lung disease
- pain, anxiety, or depression
- drugs that delay or disrupt sleep
- caffeine, tobacco, alcohol, and other substances that affect sleep
- a poor sleep environment or a change in sleep routine

If you can find the cause of this kind of insomnia, your symptoms should improve. But some people have insomnia that is not a side effect of medicines or a medical problem. This is called primary insomnia and it usually lasts at least one month.

Try nutrition and lifestyle changes to battle insomnia. Below are some of the foods that may help. Exercise and a relaxing nighttime routine also help promote sleep. If those don't work within a few weeks, get your doctor's help.

Nutrient	What it does	Food source
melatonin	regulates sleep cycle	oats cherries
tryptophan	converted to melatonin to regulate sleep cycle	spinach eggs crab
niacin	helps pineal gland produce melatonin	mushrooms nectarines tuna
vitamin B6	helps pineal gland produce melatonin	avocados carrots bananas

Irritable bowel syndrome

Irritable bowel syndrome (IBS) can certainly make you irritable. This common digestive disorder, which affects the large intestine, can cause abdominal cramping, bloating, and a change in bowel habits. Some people with IBS have constipation, while some have diarrhea. Others alternate between constipation and diarrhea. Although IBS can cause a great deal of discomfort and disrupt your life, it does not harm the intestines.

No one knows the exact cause of IBS, which strikes more women than men, and there is no specific test for it. However, your doctor may run tests to make sure you don't have other, more serious conditions. These tests include stool sampling tests, blood tests, and X-rays. Your doctor may also perform a colonoscopy or a test called a sigmoidoscopy, which examines your rectum and lower colon.

Most people diagnosed with IBS can control their symptoms with diet, stress management, and medicine. Some people believe eating foods with processed sugars and simple carbohydrates — milk, refined flour, corn syrup — causes IBS to flare up. They won't touch these foods with a 10-foot pole. Keep a journal of what you eat and what symptoms follow to figure out which are the most dangerous foods for your bowel.

Nutrient	What it does	Food source
fiber	absorbs water in the intestines to prevent diarrhea	whole-wheat bread brown rice oatmeal
probiotic bacteria	live active cultures such as acidophilus restore proper bacterial balance in intestines	yogurt fermented milk
water	helps ease fiber smoothly through digestive tract	

Kidney stones

■ ■

Sometimes big pain comes in small packages. A kidney stone, a solid pellet of material that forms in your kidney from substances in your urine, may be as small as a grain of sand or as large as a pearl. It can also feel like a boulder.

While most kidney stones pass out of the body without help from a doctor, sometimes a stone will just not go away. It may become stuck in the urinary tract, block the flow of urine, and cause excruciating pain. If you experience any of the following symptoms, you may need to see a doctor.

- extreme pain in your back or side that will not go away
- blood in your urine
- fever and chills
- vomiting
- urine that smells bad or looks cloudy
- a burning feeling when you urinate

Tests help determine if you have a kidney stone, and rule out other conditions. You may need painkillers or even noninvasive surgery to treat the problem. What you eat and drink influences kidney stone formation. Drink plenty of fluids, but cut back on salt and protein. You should also try to get more of these helpful nutrients into your diet.

Nutrient	What it does	Food source
calcium	blocks absorption of dietary oxalates, which can form stones	milk yogurt cheese sardines
magnesium	helps your body recycle wastes so they don't form stones	oatmeal wheat bran spinach black beans
potassium	increases level of citrate in urine	bananas tomatoes cherries
water	dilutes urine, washes away chemicals before they form stones	

Macular degeneration

■ ■

Macular degeneration, or age-related macular degeneration (AMD), destroys your sharp, central vision, the kind you use to see objects clearly and do tasks such as reading and driving. AMD kills the cells in the macula, the part of your eye that lets you see fine detail.

In some cases, this disease advances so slowly you may not notice much change in your vision. In other people, the disease progresses quickly and may lead to vision loss in both eyes. In fact, it's a leading cause of vision loss in people over the age of 60.

Regular comprehensive eye exams can catch AMD before it causes vision loss. Treatment can slow the damage, but it won't restore your vision.

Try to eat foods with plenty of these nutrients to lower your risk and reduce the damage of AMD.

Nutrient	What it does	Food source
lutein	works with zeaxanthin to filter UV light, stop oxidative damage	spinach kiwi avocados broccoli honeydew melon
vitamin C	slows AMD by stopping oxidative damage	citrus fruits sweet bell peppers broccoli
zeaxanthin	antioxidant that works with lutein	egg yolk orange bell peppers
zinc	found in retina of eye where it helps in chemical reactions	red meat crab wheat bran spinach black beans

Memory loss

■ ■

Some people get more forgetful with age. It may take longer to learn new things, remember familiar names and words, or find your glasses.

These are usually signs of mild forgetfulness and aren't worrisome. Serious memory lapses affect your ability to do everyday activities like drive a car, shop, or handle money. Signs of serious memory problems include:

- asking the same questions over and over again.
- becoming lost in places you know well.
- being unable to follow directions.
- getting very confused about time, people, and places.
- not taking care of yourself, such as eating poorly, not bathing, or being unsafe.

See a doctor if you are worried about your memory lapses or those of a loved one. You also can do many things to make your memory last. Having a hobby, spending time with friends, exercising, and eating well with foods like these can all help keep your mind sharp.

Nutrient	What it does	Food source
antioxidant vitamins (vitamins C and E, beta carotene)	clean up oxidative damage in brain cells	blueberries Brussels sprouts kiwi
carbohydrates	provide energy for the brain to function	oatmeal wheat bran brown rice
epicatechin	flavenol that improves brain blood flow	grapes blueberries chocolate
iron	helps form neurotransmitters to carry messages in brain	quinoa leeks beans cereals
monounsaturated fatty acids (MUFAs)	help form membranes in brain	almonds avocados walnuts

Migraines

■ ■ ■ ■ ■ ■ ■ ■ ■ ■ ■ ■ ■ ■ ■ ■

A migraine is a very painful and miserable type of headache. If you get a migraine, you'll have a pulsing or throbbing pain in one part of your head. You may also experience nausea, vomiting, dizziness, and a high sensitivity to light and sound.

Some people can even tell when they are about to have a migraine because they see flashing lights or zigzag lines or they temporarily lose their vision. Other people may suspect a migraine is coming after they encounter something that commonly causes migraines. Many things can trigger a migraine, including:

- anxiety
- stress
- lack of food or sleep
- exposure to light
- hormonal changes in women

Doctors used to believe migraines were linked to the opening and narrowing of blood vessels in the head. Now they believe brain chemistry and other factors may play a bigger role.

Drugs can help prevent migraine attacks or relieve symptoms of attacks when they happen. Lifestyle changes and nutrition may help prevent future migraines.

Nutrient	What it does	Food source
magnesium	deficiency may cause migraines	oatmeal sweet potatoes
melatonin	regulates sleep cycle to prevent onset of a migraine	oats cherries sweet corn
omega-3 fatty acids	reduce number and intensity of migraines	flaxseed salmon herring
riboflavin	reduces number and severity of migraines	spelt milk eggs

Osteoarthritis

■ ■

Getting old is a pain — especially when you have osteoarthritis. Osteoarthritis, the most common form of arthritis, often strikes older people. It can also make your life miserable.

Sometimes called degenerative joint disease, osteoarthritis mostly affects cartilage, the hard but slippery tissue that covers the ends of bones where they meet to form a joint. Healthy cartilage allows bones to glide over one another. It also absorbs energy from the shock of physical movement.

In osteoarthritis, the surface layer of cartilage breaks down and wears away. This allows bones under the cartilage to rub together, causing pain, swelling, and loss of motion of the joint. Over time, the joint may lose its normal shape. Your back, hips, knees, big toe, fingers, and base of your thumb are the most common targets of osteoarthritis, but it can affect any joint.

A combination of pain medication, physical therapy, and weight loss to decrease stress on your weight-bearing joints can help treat osteoarthritis. In serious cases, surgery may also be an option.

Controlling your weight can lessen your risk for osteoarthritis. If you are obese, losing just 11 pounds can slash your risk in half. In addition, some nutrients may offer protection.

Nutrient	What it does	Food source
boron	regulates how you use calcium and magnesium, plus it helps with vitamin D use	tomatoes raisins cherries grape juice almonds
vitamin C	helps your body manufacture collagen, a key protein in connective tissues, cartilage, and tendons	sweet peppers broccoli kiwi cherries limes nectarines
vitamin D	necessary for healthy cartilage	mushrooms, sardines

Osteoporosis

■ ■ ■ ■ ■ ■ ■ ■ ■ ■ ■ ■ ■ ■ ■ ■ ■ ■ ■ ■

People once thought a shrunken, stooped posture was a natural part of aging, but the real culprit is usually osteoporosis.

Your skeleton constantly rebuilds itself. First, cells called osteoclasts clean out between 10 and 30 percent of old bone each year. Then cells called osteoblasts form new bone. They make it from the collagen your body produces and the phosphorous and calcium you get from food.

As you age, you lose bone faster than you make it. Your bone density suffers, meaning your bones become weaker and less solid. This, in turn, makes bones more likely to fracture or break. Women lose the most bone during the first few years after menopause, but bone loss affects men as well.

Osteoporosis is the major underlying cause of fractures in post-menopausal women and the elderly, and it develops silently. You may only discover you have it when you fracture your hip or wrist during a minor bump. Little fractures in your spine may gradually reduce your height and make your posture stooped.

You can prevent this disease as well as slow its development by taking up walking, gardening, or other weight-bearing exercises to help preserve bone. Combine exercise with the right foods for the most amazing results.

Nutrient	What it does	Food source
calcium	builds skeleton to keep bones strong	milk yogurt sardines
potassium	helps prevent calcium loss	bananas honeydew melon
vitamin C	helps build collagen, an important connective tissue	red peppers grapefruit blueberries broccoli
vitamin D	helps bones store calcium, needed for bone growth	salmon sardines mushrooms
vitamin K	allows blood to clot; in the form of vitamin K2, prevents fractures	Brussels sprouts cabbage avocados lettuce

Prostate cancer

■ ■

Although it is rare in men under age 40, prostate cancer is the third most common cause of cancer deaths in men of all ages. As you may recall, the prostate is the gland below a man's bladder that wraps around the urethra, the passageway that guides urine out of the body.

Symptoms of prostate cancer may include:

- problems passing urine, such as pain, difficulty starting or stopping the stream, or dribbling
- frequent urination
- low back pain
- pain with ejaculation

The level of a substance called prostate specific antigen (PSA) is often high in men with prostate cancer, so doctors check the level of PSA as a way to screen for prostate cancer. Since the PSA test became common, most prostate cancers are found before they cause symptoms. But be aware that PSA can also be high with other prostate conditions.

Nutrition and lifestyle can help you prevent prostate cancer. However, the right prostate cancer treatment often depends on how serious the cancer has become. Treatment may include surgery, radiation therapy, chemotherapy, and control of hormones that affect the cancer.

Nutrient	What it does	Food source
fiber	binds sex hormones to remove them from body	whole-wheat bread, wheat bran, figs flaxseed
lycopene	works as a powerful antioxidant against free radicals	tomatoes, watermelon sweet red peppers grapefruit
omega-3 fatty acids (DHA and EPA from fish)	may lower risk for prostate cancer	salmon sardines trout
selenium	boosts immunity, lowers testosterone level, may kill cancer cells	Brazil nuts mushrooms, shrimp, salmon, oatmeal
vitamin E	works with selenium to boost immunity	spinach, almonds, asparagus

Rheumatoid arthritis

■ ■

Rheumatoid arthritis (RA) is an inflammatory disease you develop when your immune system attacks your joints. Experts don't understand why this happens, but they do know the consequences.

Rogue molecules cause the cushioning cartilage to break down, and the result is throbbing, warm, stiff, swollen joints. Over time, it even damages your bones. RA is more common in women and has several special features that make it different from other kinds of arthritis. For example, RA generally strikes matching joints, like both hands or both knees. People with RA may feel tired, have occasional fevers, and generally not feel well. And unlike osteoarthritis, morning stiffness from RA usually lasts more than an hour.

RA affects people differently, though. For some, it lasts only a few months or a couple of years, then goes away without causing much damage. People with mild or moderate forms of the disease go through periods of worsening symptoms, called flares, and periods in which they feel better, called remissions. Still others have a severe form that is active most of the time, lasts for years, and leads to serious joint damage and disability.

Nutrient	What it does	Food source
anthocyanins	block enzymes in body that cause inflammation and pain	cherries blueberries red grapes cranberries
copper	acts as anti-inflammatory to reduce symptoms	quinoa crab mushrooms spinach
omega-3 fatty acids	reduce inflammation to ease pain	salmon flaxseed
vitamin E	works as antioxidant to strengthen immunity	sunflower seeds almonds avocados

Sinusitis

■ ■ ■ ■ ■ ■ ■ ■ ■ ■ ■ ■ ■

If you're fed up with that swollen, achy feeling in your forehead, and your cold or hay fever seems to have lasted far longer than usual, you might have sinusitis.

Your sinuses are hollow air spaces inside the bones surrounding your nose. Sinuses produce mucus, which drains into the nose. Unfortunately, swelling in your nose can block the sinuses and cause pain and infection. When your sinuses get infected or inflamed, you have sinusitis.

Sinusitis can be acute or chronic. The acute version lasts less than four weeks while chronic sinusitis lingers longer. Acute sinusitis often starts as a cold or hay fever, but then it turns into an infection. Allergies, pollutants, nasal problems, and certain diseases can also cause sinusitis.

Symptoms of sinusitis can include fever, weakness, fatigue, cough, and congestion. You may also have postnasal drip — mucus drainage in the back of your throat. Treatments for sinusitis include antibiotics, decongestants, and pain relievers. Saline nasal sprays, vaporizers, or applying heating pads to the inflamed area can also help.

Nutrient	What it does	Food source
antioxidants (vitamin A, vitamin C, beta carotene, glutathione)	neutralize free radicals to beef up immune system and prevent infections	asparagus avocados honeydew melon sweet potatoes carrots
bromelain	loosens mucus and suppresses coughing	fresh pineapple
probiotic bacteria	live active cultures such as *Lactobacillus GG* restore proper bacterial balance in sinuses	yogurt drinks
water	moistens mucous membranes so sinuses drain properly	

Skin cancer

■ ■ ■ ■ ■ ■ ■ ■ ■ ■ ■ ■ ■ ■ ■ ■ ■

Skin cancer is the most common form of cancer in the United States. The two most common types are basal cell cancer and squamous cell cancer. These usually form on the head, face, neck, hands, and arms. Another type of skin cancer, melanoma, is more dangerous but less common.

Anyone can get skin cancer, but it is more common in people who:

- spend a lot of time in the sun or have been sunburned.
- have light-colored skin, hair, and eyes.
- have a family member with skin cancer.
- are older than age 50.

Because the sun's ultraviolet (UVA and UVB) rays promote cancer-causing changes in your skin, learning sun safe practices is one way to protect yourself. Another way is to know the signs of skin cancer. A mole that is oddly shaped, strangely colored, or unusually large may be a sign of skin cancer, especially if it grows. That's why you should check your skin regularly. You should also have your doctor check any suspicious skin markings and any changes in the way your skin looks. These steps can help you find the cancer early — the stage when cancer is most likely to be treated successfully. Catching cancer early may also prevent certain types of skin cancer cells from spreading to other parts of your body.

Nutrient	What it does	Food source
astaxanthin	destroys free radicals to prevent cell damage from UV light	salmon shrimp
catechins	work as antioxidants to prevent sun damage	green tea
d-limonene	shrinks tumors, may prevent squamous cell cancer	grapefruit (especially the peel) lemons oranges
monounsaturated fatty acids (MUFAs)	prevent oxidative damage from sun	almonds avocados walnuts

Stress

■ ■ ■ ■ ■ ■ ■ ■ ■

Everyone experiences stress sometimes. Having to speak in public, taking an important test, or going on a first date may trigger it. Stress can also come from your job, bills, and family. What causes stress for you may not be stressful for someone else. But when stress strikes, you know it. Your adrenaline starts pumping, and your body revs up to handle the crisis. Your heart may pound, your hands may sweat, or your mouth may feel dry.

Sometimes stress can be helpful by spurring you to meet a deadline or get things done. But long-term stress can take its toll on your health. Over time, stress that keeps your body on the alert can lead to wear and tear. Chronic stress may weaken your immune system and raise your risk of health problems. Research has linked stress to type 2 diabetes, irritable bowel syndrome, cancer, high blood pressure, heart disease, and depression.

If you have chronic stress, the best way to deal with it is to take care of the underlying problem. Counseling can help you find ways to relax and calm down. Some stress-busting strategies include getting a massage, taking a vacation, gardening, or listening to music. Medicines may also help. Even eating the right foods can help put your mind at ease.

Nutrient	What it does	Food source
complex carbohydrates	stimulate brain to make serotonin, a feel-good chemical	oatmeal whole-grain bread brown rice, spelt
folate	helps brain process dopamine and serotonin for relaxation	black beans, spinach, asparagus, cabbage
tryptophan	calms anxiety by helping form serotonin in the brain	crab, eggs, milk, shrimp
vitamin B12	helps make neurotransmitters to carry messages in brain	crab, salmon, tuna, turkey
vitamin C	needed to make serotonin in the brain	sweet bell peppers, kiwi, artichokes

Ulcers

A peptic ulcer, also called a gastric ulcer or duodenal ulcer, is a sore in the lining of your stomach or your duodenum, the first part of your small intestine.

People once thought peptic ulcers were caused by stress or spicy foods. Surprisingly, the real culprit is usually a bacterium called *Heliobacter pylori (H. pylori)*.

Your stomach and small intestine are protected from acidic digestive juices by a special lining. In people infected with *H. pylori,* the bacteria weaken this protective lining and allow digestive juices to eat into your stomach or small intestine, creating a painful ulcer. The good news is these ulcers can be treated with antibiotics and, in most cases, cured.

Peptic ulcers can also result from the long-term use of nonsteroidal anti-inflammatory drugs (NSAIDs) like aspirin and ibuprofen. Because they block enzymes that help protect the lining of your gut, NSAIDs quadruple your risk of getting an ulcer, especially a stomach ulcer.

Avoiding tobacco and alcohol can help you avoid aggravating ulcers. Certain compounds in food can also fight off *H. pylori* infections, helping to prevent and treat peptic ulcers.

Nutrient	What it does	Food source
allicin	kills *H. pylori*	garlic (chopped or crushed)
glutamine	helps ulcers heal	cabbage crab
proanthocyanidins	keep bacteria from attaching to stomach lining	cranberries blueberries grapes
sulforaphane	kills *H. pylori*	broccoli broccoli sprouts

Urinary tract infections

■ ■ ■ ■ ■ ■ ■ ■ ■ ■ ■ ■ ■ ■ ■ ■ ■ ■ ■ ■

Infections of the urinary tract (UTIs) are the second most common type of infection in the body. You may have a UTI if you notice:

- pain or burning when you use the bathroom.
- fever, tiredness, or shakiness.
- an urge to use the bathroom often.
- pressure in your lower belly.
- urine that smells bad or looks cloudy or reddish.

Bacteria are the villains behind UTIs. In fact, harmful bacteria from your stool sometimes manage to sneak into the urethra, the opening where urine exits your body. From there, they may spread to your bladder. Urinating helps wash these bacteria out of the urinary tract, so anything that makes you urinate less raises your odds of a UTI.

If you think you have a UTI, see your doctor. She can tell whether you have a UTI by testing a sample of your urine. Treatment with medicines to kill the infection will make it better, often in one or two days. The following nutrients will go a long way toward helping you avoid an infection.

Nutrient	What it does	Food source
proanthocyanidins	keep bacteria from attaching to urinary tract lining	cranberries, cranberry juice, blueberries, grapes, lignonberries
probiotic bacteria	live active cultures prevent growth of disease-causing bacteria, keep environment acidic	fermented milk yogurt
vitamin C	makes urine more acidic to hinder growth of bacteria	grapefruit, kiwi cherries, sweet peppers
water	flushes bacteria from urinary tract	

Weight gain

■ ■ ■ ■ ■ ■ ■ ■ ■ ■ ■ ■ ■ ■ ■ ■ ■ ■ ■ ■

If you are overweight, you are not alone. In the United States, 66 percent of adults are overweight or obese. Fortunately, achieving a healthy weight can help you control your cholesterol, blood pressure, and blood sugar. It might also help you avoid weight-related diseases, such as heart disease, diabetes, arthritis, and some cancers.

Eating too much or not getting enough physical activity make many people overweight. To lose weight, you must use more calories than you eat. But don't bother with quick weight-loss schemes or starvation diets. Believe it or not, they can actually make you fat. When you're hungry, your body's natural response is to compensate by overeating. Then the pounds come right back on. Instead, gradually adopt healthy habits.

- A practical weight-control strategy might include these steps.
- Choose low-fat, low-calorie foods.
- Eat smaller portions.
- Drink water instead of sugary drinks.
- Be physically active.
- Don't skip breakfast.

Add more bulk to your diet in the form of fiber. You can trim your waistline just by switching from high-glycemic white bread to tasty whole-wheat bread. Here are more foods that can help you maintain a healthy weight.

Nutrient	What it does	Food source
calcium	signals body to burn fat rather than storing it	low-fat milk, yogurt kale
catechins	slow carbohydrate digestion by blocking digestive enzymes	green tea
fiber	adds bulk to food so it fills you up faster, for longer periods; stabilizes blood sugar	wheat bran, oatmeal black beans, figs, fennel whole-wheat bread
naringin	blocks digestive enzymes in small intestine	grapefruit
water	fills you up; may raise metabolism to burn more calories	

Yeast infections
■ ■

Don't panic if your doctor says you have candidiasis or moniliasis. He's just saying you have a yeast infection.

Candida is the scientific name for yeast. It is a fungus that lives almost everywhere, including in your body. Usually your immune system keeps yeast under control. But if you are sick or taking antibiotics, it can multiply and cause an infection in one or more parts of your body. Some people think a diet with lots of sugar can encourage yeast infections. In fact, repeated yeast infections can even be a sign of diabetes.

Yeast infections affect different parts of the body in different ways.

- Thrush is a yeast infection that causes white patches in your mouth. Sometime thrush can spread to your esophagus, the tube that takes food from your mouth to your stomach. Then the infection is called esophagitis, and you may find swallowing difficult or painful.
- Women can get vaginal yeast infections, causing itchiness, pain, and discharge.
- Yeast infections of the skin cause itching and rashes.
- Yeast infections in your bloodstream can be life threatening.

Antifungal medicines eliminate yeast infections in most people. Certain foods can help as well.

Nutrient	What it does	Food source
probiotic bacteria	live active cultures maintain proper bacterial balance to prevent yeast infection	yogurt fermented milk
vitamin C	increases acidity of vagina, making it unfriendly for yeast	broccoli sweet bell peppers kiwi honeydew melon

Index

■ ■ ■ ■ ■ ■ ■ ■ ■

I

K

L

Niacin
  for cholesterol 175
  for insomnia 346
  for vision 331
  in mushrooms 95
Night blindness 73-74
Nitrosamines 119, 252
Nut butters 277
NutraSweet. *See* Aspartame
Nutrient-dense foods 2, 28
Nutrition Facts panel 29
Nuts. *See also* Almonds, Pistachios,
  and Walnuts
  allergies to 284
  for weight loss 283

O

Oat groats 230
Oatmeal 228-232
Oil
  amaranth 222
  coconut 272
  comparisons 277
  flaxseed 276
  olive 178
  palm 272
  sunflower 287
Oleocanthal 179
Olives 176-180
Omega-3 fatty acids 12
  for allergies 342
  for Alzheimer's disease 327
  for arthritis 355
  for cancer 53, 330, 354
  for depression 335
  for diabetes 336
  for high blood pressure 344

  for migraines 351
  in fish 295
Omega-6 fatty acids 11
Onions, spring 107-110
Oolong tea 25
Oral cancer, citrus fruits for 171
Orange juice, for weight loss 213-
  214
Organic food 55
Organosulfur compounds 9
Osteoarthritis (OA) 352. *See also*
  Arthritis
  bok choy for 53
  onions for 108
  pomegranates for 198
Osteocalcin 50, 63
Osteoporosis 353
  artichokes for 44-45
  asparagus for 50
  avocados for 132
  bananas for 136
  berries for 201-202
  Brussels sprouts for 63
  calcium for 41
  copper for 236
  dried plums for 193-194
  honeydew melon for 164-165
  magnesium for 45
  manganese for 251
  menopause and 263-264
  oxalates and 60
  pineapple for 187
  plantains for 191
  potassium for 165
  sardines for 300-301
  starfruit for 209-210
  vitamin C for 45, 165
  vitamin D for 41
  vitamin K for 44, 50